European School of Oncology

Monographs

Series Editor: U. Veronesi

The European School of Oncology gratefully acknowledges sponsorship for the production of this monograph received from SmithKline Beecham.

Springer

Berlin
Heidelberg
New York
Barcelona
Budapest
Hong Kong
London
Milan
Paris
Santa Clara
Singapore
Tokyo

M. Tonato (Ed.)

Antiemetics in the Supportive Care of Cancer Patients

With 3 Figures and 28 Tables

Springer

Maurizio Tonato, M.D.
Medical Oncology Division
Policlinico Monteluce
Via Brunamonti
06122 Perugia, Italy

Library of Congress Cataloging-in-Publication Data
Antiemetics in the supportive care of cancer patients / M. Tonato (ed.).
(Monographs / European School of Oncology)
Includes bibliographical references.
ISBN-13: 978-3-642-80242-3 e-ISBN-13: 978-3-642-80240-9
DOI: 10.1007/978-3-642-80240-9
1. Antineoplastic agents--Side effects--Chemotherapy. 2. antiemetics. 3. Nausea--Chemotherapy.
I. Tonato, M. (Maurizio) II. Series: Monographs (European School of Oncology)
[DNLM: 1. Neoplasms--drug therapy. 2. Antiemetics--therapeutic use. QZ 267 A6295 1996]
RC271.C5A675 1996 616.99'4061--dc20

Softcover reprint of the hardcover 1st edition 1996

Typesetting: Camera ready by editor
SPIN: 10132192 19/3133 - 5 4 3 2 1 0 – Printed on acid-free paper

Foreword

The European School of Oncology came into existence to respond to a need for information, education and training in the field of the diagnosis and treatment of cancer. There are two main reasons why such an initiative was considered necessary. Firstly, the teaching of oncology requires a rigorously multidisciplinary approach which is difficult for the Universities to put into practice since their system is mainly disciplinary orientated. Secondly, the rate of technological development that impinges on the diagnosis and treatment of cancer has been so rapid that it is not an easy task for medical faculties to adapt their curricula flexibly.

With its residential courses for organ pathologies and the seminars on new techniques (laser, monoclonal antibodies, imaging techniques etc.) or on the principal therapeutic controversies (conservative or mutilating surgery, primary or adjuvant chemotherapy, radiotherapy alone or integrated), it is the ambition of the European School of Oncology to fill a cultural and scientific gap and, thereby, create a bridge between the University and Industry and between these two and daily medical practice.

One of the more recent initiatives of ESO has been the institution of permanent study groups, also called task forces, where a limited number of leading experts are invited to meet once a year with the aim of defining the state of the art and possibly reaching a consensus on future developments in specific fields of oncology.

The ESO Monograph series was designed with the specific purpose of disseminating the results of these study group meetings, and providing concise and updated reviews of the topic discussed.

It was decided to keep the layout relatively simple, in order to restrict the costs and make the monographs available in the shortest possible time, thus overcoming a common problem in medical literature: that of the material being outdated even before publication.

Umberto Veronesi
Chairman Scientific Committee
European School of Oncology

Contents

Introduction

Maurizio Tonato

Medical Oncology Division, Policlinico Monteluce, Via Brunamonti, 06122 Perugia, Italy

From a cancer patient's point of view, nausea and vomiting are the most distressing complications of chemotherapy, but they can also be caused by a variety of other conditions that one should always consider before beginning antiemetic treatment. Nausea and vomiting affect very negatively the psychological status, nutritional balance, social relationships, and ultimately, quality of life of the patient. Furthermore, when nausea and vomiting are caused by chemotherapy, and this is the most frequent situation in cancer patients, their intensity and persistence can bring the patient to a refusal of treatment, even if it is potentially curative. Thus, every effort should be made to clarify the real causes of nausea and vomiting and to treat these symptoms adequately.

During the last decade, considerable progress has been made in the pharmacological treatment of chemotherapy-induced emesis. Before the 1980s, emesis was considered by oncologists an almost unavoidable consequence of cancer chemotherapy, and only a few clinical trials on its prevention were planned and conducted. The introduction in clinical practice of cisplatin, which causes emesis in the majority of patients when used without a valid treatment, and its wide use in the treatment of advanced cancer, stimulated studies on antiemetic therapy that have made possible considerable advances in the prevention of chemotherapy-induced emesis.

This progress was achieved through the recognition of different emetic problems (acute, delayed, and anticipatory emesis) and clarification of some aspects of the neuropharmacology of nausea and vomiting, identification of effective antiemetic agents, used alone or in combination, and the adoption of sound methodology in clinical research. Notwithstanding these advances, emesis remains a critical problem in cancer patients, and basic and clinical research still must go far to achieve the ideal goal, that is, the complete control of such symptoms in every cancer patient.

The scientific production concerning antiemetics has been impressively large in the last ten to fifteen years, so the need for a manual on antiemetics comes only from the possibility of having at hand an up-to-date, comprehensive, easy to consult text. This is what I have tried to accomplish by bringing together various experts in different aspects of antiemetic research so as to have all the area properly covered.

One fundamental step ahead in antiemetic research was a better understanding of the mechanisms of nausea and vomiting induced by chemotherapy. An authority in this field, P.L.R. Andrews, extensively illustrates in the first chapter the different aspects of induction and control of emesis from an experimental point of view that also has important clinical implications.

After the discussion of the essential pharmacology of antiemetics by S. Grunberg, and the presentation of methodological issues by E. Ballatori, the problem of antiemetic treatment of the most emetogenic chemotherapy, cisplatin, is presented by P.H.M. De Mulder and J. Verweij. The introduction of the new antiserotoninergic drugs made possible important progress with complete protection in approximately 80% of cases, although some aspects (which antiserotoninergic drugs should be used, and at which dose) should be better clarified in the near future.

Treatment of emesis caused by chemotherapy other than cisplatin has a relevant role in clinical practice because of the extensive utilisation in settings like the adjuvant treatments. M. Martin and E. Díaz-Rubio present the up-to-date results and standards of treatment in this area.

As control of acute vomiting improved it became clear that virtually all patients given high-dose cisplatin had nausea and vomiting that started after the first 24 hours. This was defined as delayed emesis, a phenomenon that affects quality of life very negatively. M.S. Aapro gives an overview of the treatments that are used and depicts the chances for improving the results that nowadays are not satisfactory.

Radiotherapy is also an important cause of emesis, especially when the upper abdomen is irradiated or when radiotherapy is used as total-body irradiation (TBI), as in the conditioning regimens for bone marrow transplantation. The results and perspectives of antiemetic therapy in this area are presented by T.J. Priestman.

Treatment of a very common and feared symptom of cancer, pain, can induce nausea and vomiting. The increasingly widespread use of narcotic analgesics in cancer patients raises the problem, here illustrated by F. Roila, of adequately treating this side-effect. The antiemetic treatment of paediatric patients with their peculiar susceptibility to some side-effects with the use of certain drugs, e.g. metoclopramide, is presented by R.F. Stevens.

The chapter by S. Wilkinson highlights the role of nursing in the management of emesis, a role that is very important due to the close contact of nurses with patients and their problems.

An important issue, the cost of antiemetic therapies, is presented by V. Kirchner and M.S. Aapro, while J. Herrstedt illustrates the possibilities of alternative treatments.

The last chapter sheds light on the future of antiemetics and on the possibility of solving the still pending problems. This is presented by A. Del Favero, E. Ballatori and F. Roila, my friends and colleagues in the Perugia team, the core of the Italian Group for Antiemetic Research that has accomplished so much in the area of antiemetics.

Coordination of research efforts in these areas will certainly lead to improved remedies and improved quality of life for our patients. With all the authors being so experienced and esteemed in their field I am sure that this manual on antiemetics will be a valid instrument for everyone involved in cancer therapy.

Acknowledgement

First of all I would like to thank all authors of this monograph for their commitment to the project. I am also grateful to the ESO staff for their help in organising this task force. A special mention to Marije de Jager for her editorial support in Milan, and to my secretary Patricia Boyce here in Perugia.

The Mechanism of Emesis Induced by Chemotherapy and Radiotherapy

Paul L.R. Andrews

Department of Physiology, St George's Hospital Medical School, Cranmer Terrace, London SW17 0RE, United Kingdom

Nausea and vomiting are two of the side-effects of major concern to patients undergoing palliative or curative chemo- or radiotherapy for cancer and both have a variety of deleterious effects on the patient's quality of life during treatment. Vomiting itself places a considerable physical stress on the body in patients who may already be weakened by their disease and any concomitant surgery. Tearing of the oesophagus (Mallory-Weiss Syndrome) and herniation of the stomach may occur, as can abdominal muscle strain, purpura, fatigue and even fracture of ribs if the vomiting is particularly violent [1]. The main danger is from aspiration of vomitus, although this is considered to be a greater risk in patients vomiting during emergence from anaesthesia. Protracted vomiting has metabolic effects including alkalosis and hyponatraemia (due to loss of gastric hydrogen and sodium ions) and the difficulty in retaining food together with nausea-induced food aversion (see below) could lead to a degree of malnutrition [1]. The importance of the psychological effects of nausea and vomiting have only been truly appreciated in recent years [2]. Vomiting is considered to be a degrading or humiliating act, particularly if it occurs in front of other patients. This should not be overlooked in the design of oncology units, not only from the aspect of the patient receiving therapy but also for those waiting. The sight of someone vomiting may itself induce emesis in susceptible individuals but the smell of vomitus which may linger is also a potent nauseogenic stimulus. The nausea accompanying chemotherapy will contribute to aversion to food and, of greater clinical significance, it plays an important role in inducing avoidance of further courses of therapy and anticipatory nausea and vomiting [3]. By preventing the induction of nausea and vomiting occurring as a result of cytostatic treatment, not only will there be direct effects to the patient of avoiding the unpleasant physical, metabolic and psychological effects, but also indirect benefits. These include a general improvement in their well-being which should improve their intrinsic ability to cope with the disease both physically and emotionally, and an increased likelihood of completing multiple-cycle therapy resulting in a reduced morbidity and mortality.

This chapter reviews our understanding of the basic mechanisms by which cytotoxic anticancer drugs and radiation induce emesis. An understanding of these mechanisms is essential for the design of rational antiemetic therapy and for interpretation of the mechanism and sites of action of the antiemetic agents.

The Clinical Problem of Nausea and Vomiting from a Biological Perspective

Whilst nausea and vomiting are most often encountered in a clinical context, it is critical to an understanding of the way in which they are induced by anticancer therapies to appreciate that they are both "natural" events contributing to the body's defensive system against accidentally ingested toxins [4]: vomiting serving to expel the toxin from the upper gastrointestinal tract and nausea to generate an aversion and hence avoidance of that cause in the future. In the context of ingestion of contaminated food these responses are "appropriate" and lead to expulsion of the toxin. However, in the context of anticancer therapy they are "inappropriate" by virtue of the fact that the "toxin" (i.e., the chemotherapy drug) is in the circulation and vomiting will thus have little effect in removing it from the body. In addition, the aversion induced may give rise to anticipatory nausea and vomiting and avoidance of further courses of therapy. The latter is of particular concern in the context of oncology where number and timing of cytotoxic drug doses or radiation fractions may be critical for optimising the antitumour effects.

To trigger nausea and vomiting all that is required is that the cytotoxic drug or radiation (both of which can be regarded as "cellular poisons") accesses and activates one or more of the systems that are presumed to have evolved for the detection of toxins in the food. Viewing the nausea and vomiting induced by anticancer therapy in this way promotes a more rational basis for understanding these side-effects and, more significantly, has provided a focus for the mechanistic studies. By considering the parallels between emesis induced in the "natural" as opposed to the "clinical" environment it becomes apparent that the best way of preventing the entire cascade of direct emetic, psychological and behavioural effects of therapy is to prevent the initial activation of the emetic inputs. In addition, this consideration clearly illustrates that optimal antiemetic therapy (irrespective of cost!) should be given at the first course of treatment and not be reserved for "failures" because of the increased probability of inducing anticipatory emetic responses and avoidance of further therapy.

General Mechanisms of Emesis

Before discussing the specific mechanisms underlying anticancer therapy-induced emesis, some of the more general aspects will be discussed, covering the mechanics of retching and vomiting, the central integration of the motor outputs and the various pathways for the induction of vomiting and nausea.

Motor Components

This section deals with the visceral and somatic motor events involved in expulsion of material or in preparation for expulsion. The gastrointestinal motility patterns which have been associated with the sensation of nausea are discussed below. The motor components can be divided into two distinct but consecutive phases: pre-ejection and ejection, which are described separately.

Pre-ejection phase

The pre-ejection phase is usually associated with the sensation of nausea and a number of indications of sympathetic nervous system activation including cold sweating, skin pallor, pupil dilation and tachycardia [5]. Salivation may also occur, probably under parasympathetic influence. Such changes are not specific to the prodromal phase of vomiting but also occur in association with pain and are best regarded as an indication of a more general autonomic arousal perhaps due to the stressful nature of nausea. Specific changes in gastrointestinal motility occur in the period immediately preceding the onset of retching and vomiting, the most notable being gastric relaxation, retrograde peristaltic activity in the small intestine and tonic longitudinal contraction of the pharyngo-oesophageal junction [6,7]. The relaxation of the proximal stomach appears to be the initial event and this occurs by vagal efferent activation of intrinsic non-adrenergic, non-cholinergic inhibitory neurones, probably using vasoactive intestinal polypeptide and nitric oxide as neurotransmitters. The lower oesophageal sphincter is also relaxed at this time. Once the proximal stomach is relaxed, a single large contraction originates in the mid-small intestine and propagates retrogradely towards the stomach. This single contraction is termed the retrograde giant contraction (RGC) and is under vagal control via the release of acetylcholine. The tonic contraction of the pharyngo-oesophageal junction occurs after the initiation of the RGC.

These motor events, although not directly responsible for the expulsion of vomit, are considered to have a function: the gastric relaxation will help to confine any contaminated food to the stomach and in addition may place the stomach in the most mechanically advantageous position for compression by somatic muscles; the RGC will return contaminated intestinal contents to the stomach which is the only place from which ejection can occur. In addition, it has been suggested that the alkaline intestinal secretions carried into the stomach by the RGC may help to neutralize the acid gastric contents and so reduce damage to teeth and oesophagus [8]: this could be further assisted by the enhanced salivary secretion and swallowing often reported to occur prior to vomiting; the tonic pharyngo-oesophageal contraction is suggested to shorten the intra-abdominal segment of the oesophagus, reduce the acute angle between the stomach and the oesophagus (valve of His) and make the proximal stomach into a funnel [8]. All of these events will facilitate the movement of gastric contents into the oesophagus during the expulsive phase.

The gastrointestinal motor events are an integral component of the normal vomiting reflex but if their occurrence is prevented experimentally by cutting the abdominal vagi then retching and vomiting can still occur [6,8]. However, when the vagi are intact, these events are carefully integrated with the somatic events such that retching will not begin until the RGC has reached the stomach.

Ejection phase

In contrast to the pre-ejection phase which predominantly involves the autonomic nervous system, the ejection phase is under somatic control and is characterised by retching and vomiting with expulsion only occurring during the latter. The ejection of gastric contents is brought about by compression of the stomach by contraction of the anterior abdominal muscles and diaphragm, however, electromyographic studies have revealed some subtle differences between retching and vomiting [9,10]. During retching the entire diaphragm contracts, the lower oesophageal sphincter is relaxed and vomitus enters the oesophagus. The upper oesophageal sphincter is relaxed during each retch but surprisingly there is no oral expulsion of vomitus [6]. The reason for this appears to be twofold. Firstly, during vomiting in contrast to retching, the peri-oesophageal portion of the diaphragm relaxes and it is thought that this relaxation removes the last barrier preventing bulk expulsion of material. Secondly, recent studies in the dog indicate that during vomiting but not retching there may be an oesophago-pharyngeal retrograde contraction which promotes expulsion of material. This is coupled with a powerful contraction of the geniohyoideus muscle which further opens the already relaxed upper oesophageal sphincter [6].

From the above description it can be seen that approaches to antiemesis targeted at blocking the motor components of emesis will be unsuccessful. Experimental animal studies have shown that the gastrointestinal motility changes are not essential for retching or vomiting and as both of these involve muscles essential for normal respiration, blockade of their actions (e.g. by curare derivatives) is impracticable.

Central Integration of the Motor Components

The motor components of emetic reflex involve the careful integration of the visceral and somatic responses described above, together with the complex series of changes in behaviour and sensation which constitute nausea. They must also be coordinated with respiration which involves many of the same muscle groups. Indeed, the imperative to resume normal respiration may be one of the factors that regulates the number of retches in a burst [11]. The coordination of the motor components of the vomiting reflex occurs in the brainstem. This is the region where there is convergence between the abdominal vagal afferents, the outputs from the area postrema and descending inputs from higher areas of the CNS (e.g. amygdala). There has been considerable speculation over the years about whether there is a single anatomical site which could be described as the "vomiting centre" [12]. At present this issue has not been resolved but there are three structures which have been implicated.

a) The nucleus tractus solitarius. This nucleus, located dorsally in the caudal brainstem, is the major integrative nucleus for visceral information and sends outputs to the major motor nuclei (e.g. dorsal motor vagal nucleus) involved in emesis [13]. In addition, its ventral region forms the so-called "dorsal respiratory group" of neurones which, together with the "ventral respiratory group", are involved in regulating the output to the diaphragm, intercostal and abdominal muscles.
b) The electrical stimulation studies of Wang and Borison [see 12 for refs] identified a region in the dorsolateral border of the lateral reticular formation from which emesis could occasionally be induced and more often individual prodromal components (e.g. licking). They proposed that this region was

the vomiting centre. On neuroanatomical grounds Mehler [14] proposed that the parvicellular reticular formation was the location of the emetic coordinating mechanism.

c) The Bötzinger complex of neurones in the region of the retrofacial nucleus has attracted attention recently as a possible site of the emetic pattern generator based mainly on lesion studies [15,16], and although the results are suggestive of such a role, more definitive electrophysiological studies need to be undertaken.

The current view is that there is unlikely to be a single anatomical site which could be called the "vomiting centre" but that the patterning of the emetic response is a higher expression or product of the interactions between a network of neurones (i.e., a "local" circuit is the central pattern generator for vomiting [vomiting centre]). This view is consistent with the experimental observation that individual components of the emetic response may be elicited by electrical stimulation of brainstem structures more readily than the entire emetic response. From what is known of the anatomical connectivity and physiology of the nucleus tractus solitarius it is clear that much of this network is likely to reside in this nucleus with the output going to the visceral (e.g. DMVN) and somatic (e.g. Bötzinger complex) output nuclei. It is likely that there is some provision for feedback (e.g. efferent copy) between the outputs and the integrating mechanism (e.g. NTS) to regulate the number of retches and vomits, their individual magnitude and the transition point between retching and vomiting.

Although the exact nature of the "vomiting centre" is not known, the term provides a convenient shorthand for the anatomical substrate involved in the integrative processes and motor outputs for emesis.

Regarding the vomiting centre in this way has implications for the design of antiemetic drugs. If there is a single nucleus then it would be conceivable to target this structure but if, as is suspected, there is a network then this is a much harder problem. In addition, it must be remembered that all the motor outputs which contribute to emesis have non-emetic routine functions which could be disrupted by a drug targeted at this network. There are, however, two possibilities which may allow consideration of the brainstem network as a potential site for an antiemetic drug. Firstly, evidence is emerging that there may be an endogenous mechanism which can modulate the emetic mechanism. In brief, several studies have reported that the opiate receptor antagonist naloxone can enhance the response to a variety of central and peripherally acting emetic stimuli and some opiate receptor agonists are antiemetic [17]. These studies suggest that some critical component of the central emetic pathway is under tonic suppression by an opiate mechanism. Access to this mechanism could provide a "universal" antiemetic. Secondly, it is possible that co-transmission (two transmitters released from one synapse) occurs within the emetic network. The emetic response is produced by a particular sequence and intensity of activation of nuclei that also have non-emetic functions. It is conceivable that in their non-emetic functions one neurotransmitter is used but for the intense activation required for emesis an additional transmitter is co-released. If this is the case then blockade of the co-transmitter alone could block emesis without interfering with non-emetic functions and perhaps nausea, which is often regarded as being caused by "low" intensity activation of the emetic pathway.

General Activation of the Emetic Pathwa

As a background to the discussion of the specific pathways and mechanisms by which cytotoxic drugs and radiation induce emesis, the general emetic pathways will be reviewed.

Area postrema

The area postrema (AP) is part of the circumventricular organ system (other examples are the subfornical organ and the OVLT) and viewed from the surface is a U-shaped structure located at the caudal extremity of the fourth ventricle. The density of neurones is quite low in comparison to other brainstem regions but the AP is highly vascularised and the capillaries are fenestrated so that it is often described as being located outside the blood-brain barrier. In addition, the ependymal cells covering the ventricular surface of the area postrema have gaps between them so that relatively large molecules in the cerebrospinal fluid can access the interstitium of the AP. These structural features suggest that the area postrema has a "chemoreceptor" function. The outputs from the AP are to the nucleus tractus solitarius and the parabrachial nucleus and via these the AP could influence a wide variety of autonomic and behavioural responses. It is worth pointing out that the AP has been implicated in a variety of functions other than emesis and these include conditioned taste aversion, food and salt intake and blood pressure regulation [18]. Thus the AP is not solely an "emetic detector", a view supported by the observation that animals lacking an emetic response have an area postrema. It is probably wiser and more accurate to describe the AP as "a chemoreceptive region" rather than "the chemoreceptor trigger zone for emesis".

In the context of emesis there are two types of stimuli to consider from the aspect of how they could activate the area postrema: emetic drugs such as apomorphine which are pharmacological receptor agonists, and cytotoxic drugs such as cisplatin. In the case of apomorphine all that is required for it to induce emesis is that dopamine D_2 receptors are present on AP neurones which are capable of activating the output of the AP to the emetic motor pathways. In addition, as dendrites from neurones in the NTS arborise into the AP, it is possible that they could provide another site at which emetic drugs could act [19]. For agents such as cisplatin the problem is more complex: if this and other cytotoxic agents had their primary emetic effect on the AP, a mechanism would need to be proposed by which they could activate the neurones and there are several possibilities.

a) Cytotoxic drugs could directly (e.g. a change in membrane ionic conductance [20]) or indirectly (e.g. modification of transmitter synthesis or degradation [20] or release via free radical generation [21]) influence either the AP neurones or specialised chemoreceptor cells (cf. carotid body glomus cells) to cause activation of emetic outputs. There is no evidence that drugs such as cisplatin bind directly to pharmacological receptors to act as agonists [22]. The difficulty is that most of the evidence for the involvement of the area postrema in emesis has been based on ablation studies rather than recordings from AP neurones, which is technically difficult. The studies of Carpenter and colleagues [23] recording from AP neurones in the dog have clearly demonstrated that neurones in the AP respond to a wide variety of neurotransmitter substances when they are applied locally, and many of these substances can induce emesis when administered systemically. Whilst these studies provide the neurophysiological correlate for the studies which have demonstrated an abolition of emesis induced by a number of pharmacological receptor agonists (e.g. apomorphine) by AP ablation, they have to date not provided equivalent support for a primary action of cytotoxic drugs at this site. One potentially important finding from the studies of Carpenter and colleagues relates to modulation of AP sensitivity. They demonstrated that the emetic threshold to apomorphine could be reduced by using phosphodiesterase inhibitors (e.g. theophylline, IBMX), which raise the intracellular levels of cAMP [23]. Although the weight of evidence favours a peripheral site as the primary one at which cytotoxic drugs act (see below), it is possible that they may have a secondary central action to reduce the threshold of the area postrema or indeed the NTS to other emetic inputs. Whilst the emphasis for studies of cytotoxic emesis has shifted away from the area postrema to the vagus and the gut mucosa, it would be unwise to forget the area postrema, particularly as 5-HT_3 receptor antagonists are not fully effective in the acute phase in all cancer patients and we do not yet have satisfactory mechanisms to explain the delayed phase.

b) Abdominal visceral afferents: The upper gastrointestinal tract is supplied with afferents from the vagus and the greater splanchnic nerves [24]. In brief, the abdominal vagal afferents signal information to the brainstem (mainly the nucleus tractus solitarius but also the area postrema) from two sets of receptor:

1) "in series" tension receptors located in the muscles signal distension and contraction of the stomach and small intestine. Over the physiological range these afferents are responsible for vago-vagal reflexes regulating motility and give rise to sensations of comfortable fullness. When the stomach or intestine are overdistended it is probably these afferents which trigger emesis.

2) "chemoreceptors" located in the mucosa signal a number of features of the luminal environment including pH, osmolarity, and temperature. In addition, the mucosal receptors respond to gentle mechanical stimulation such as that which could be produced by particulate matter brushing against the mucosa. These afferents are the ones which are involved in the emetic response to luminal hypertonic solutions and copper sulphate. The anatomical substrate for this receptor is considered to be similar to other types of chemoreceptor such as the taste buds and the carotid body, i.e., a cell which actually detects the stimulus and via the release of a neurotransmitter activates an afferent terminating in close proximity. In the case of the gut mucosal chemoreceptor, one of the detector cells is proposed to be the enterochromaffin cell releasing 5-HT and probably a number of other neuroactive agents, e.g. Substance P (see below).

The splanchnic afferents appear to be mainly involved in signalling noxious levels of distension and inflammation of the muscle and serosa. The role of these afferents in emesis is still being defined. Whilst nausea commonly accompanies intense pain, stimulation of the afferents in the greater splanchnic nerve does not induce emesis as would occur with abdominal vagal afferent stimulation. Although the splanchnic afferents do not appear to have a direct involvement in emesis, they do appear capable of modifying the response [25]. Several studies have shown that whilst section of the greater splanchnic nerves does not abolish the emetic response to cytotoxic drugs or total body radiation and indeed frequently increases the number of retches, section of the greater splanchnic nerve in combination with vagotomy often achieves better results than vagotomy alone [25,26]. At present there is no satisfactory explanation for this observation but the involvement of the splanchnic afferents requires further investigation.

Other inputs

Although the area postrema and the abdominal vagal afferents are the inputs most involved in triggering the primary emetic response to cytotoxic drugs and radiation, emesis can be induced from other sites and these are outlined here as they could have a secondary involvement:

Vestibular system: This is responsible for the emetic response to motion stimuli and sensitivity to motion sickness is one of the predisposing factors to cytotoxic drug-induced emesis (see below). Concomitant labyrinthine stimulation can modify the response to emetic stimuli acting at other sites (e.g. apomorphine on the area postrema [27]). This factor should be borne in mind if patients are moved on a trolley or wheelchair following chemo- or radiotherapy.

Taste: In some sensitive individuals gagging and emesis can be induced by unpleasant tastes, although the mechanism appears to be by association rather than primary activation of the emetic system. Some chemotherapy agents given intravenously induce a bitter or metallic taste sensation. An unpleasant smell, particularly vomit, may also induce nausea or emesis and this should be considered in the design of oncology units.

Higher CNS influences: Whilst there is little doubt that the psychological state of an individual can modify the response to an emetic agent, little is known of the central pathways mediating this response. At some point these pathways must either directly activate the vomiting centre or, more likely, the nucleus tractus solitarius to initiate the entire emetic motor programme. In man, monkey and dog, electrical stimulation of the amygdala (a region of the brain involved in emotional responses) induced emesis and in man this was accompanied by nausea [28-30]. Further support for the involvement of cerebral structures in emesis is provided by the observation that nausea and vomiting accompany some psychiatric disorders [31]. Cerebral lesions in the cat can reduce the emetic response to nitrogen mustard [32]. In addition to direct emetic effects, higher structures could also alter the sensitivity of the nucleus tractus solitarius to a variety of emetic inputs and thus provide a pathway for understanding psychological influences on emetic sensitivity.

Nausea

This is an unpleasant, but not painful, sensation associated with the desire to vomit or the feeling that vomiting is imminent. It is often associated with sensations in the throat or stomach but the degree to which these are primary or referred is unclear. Although there are few, if any, outward signs of nausea in contrast to vomiting, its clinical significance should not be underestimated. Indeed, nausea may be a more serious problem than vomiting because it tends to be continuous with increasing waves of intensity, whereas retching and vomiting occur in discrete bursts. In addition, vomiting is often followed by relief of the sensation of nausea. The mechanism underlying this has not been investigated but is most likely to be due to a release of an endorphin. The way in which the subjective sensation of nausea occurs is not known but in general stimulation of the pathways described above at levels of stimulation which do not evoke vomiting can induce nausea. This mechanism is broadly consistent with the proposed function of nausea as a warning signal that the body has been exposed to a toxin, usually contaminated food, but in this context a chemotherapeutic drug or radiation. The generation of the sensation requires projection of information from the various emetic inputs to cerebral structures. Projections of the nucleus tractus solitarius and parabrachial nucleus have been identified which could provide an anatomical substrate for such information transfer [13].

One of the difficulties in studying the mechanism underlying nausea is that, because it is a sensation (cf. retching and vomiting), it cannot be studied in animals and such studies are limited to measuring what we may recognise or interpret as "behavioural equivalents". This problem also applies to studies of pain in animals where we can only measure the response to a stimulus we consider painful (e.g. limb withdrawal to a pinch) and not the animal's perception of the stimulus. For this reason the discussion will be confined to studies in man. Attention has focussed on two areas which will be reviewed separately.

Vasopressin

Numerous studies have demonstrated that in subjects (human and animal) exposed to emetic stimuli including motion, apomorphine and cytotoxic drugs [34-39], the sensation of nausea in animals was accompanied by a large increase in plasma vasopressin (antidiuretic hormone, ADH). In the absence of nausea no large rise in vasopressin is seen and in many studies a correlation was found between vasopressin levels and symptom intensity. Similar changes in vasopressin have been observed in animals exposed to the same stimuli. Although there are many other endocrine changes associated with the prodromal phase of emesis (e.g. increase in ACTH, beta-endorphin), the increase in vasopressin is considered to be the earliest and most significant.

The greatest problem with interpretation of these vasopressin studies is whether the rise in vasopressin is the cause of nausea or is a component of the endocrine response to the stressful nature of the experience. At present it is not possible to distinguish between these two possibilities; however, it is possible that the truth lies somewhere between these two extremes. Vasopressin is not obligatory for the induction of nausea or vomiting as studies in patients with diabetes insipidus experience both when given apomorphine or ipecacuanha [35]. Motion was not studied. This study does not exclude some involvement of vasopressin in nausea and vomiting. Intravenous administration of vasopressin readily induces nausea and many of the autonomically mediated responses which accompany nausea (e.g. salivation, headache, cold extremities [39]). In the squirrel monkey a vasopressin (V-1) receptor antagonist produced a blockade of motion-induced emesis and marked reduction in symptom score [40]. These observations can to some extent be reconciled in the following speculative way. Vasopressin is initially released as part of the general stress response and as this continues, further enhanced by the sensation of nausea, vasopressin levels increase dramatically until they reach a level where they are having a direct action on the emetic system in the brainstem themselves. This facilitates the emetic effect of the primary stimulus (e.g. motion, cytotoxic drug). However, the absence of vasopressin would not necessarily prevent the occurrence of nausea but might reduce the intensity. If the emetic stimulus was mild then blockade of the effects of vasopressin could be sufficient to prevent nausea and vomiting but if it was intense then the direct emetic effects of the stimulus could still cause the full response in the absence of vasopressin.

Gastrointestinal Motility

Although the sensation of nausea is often associated with the upper gastrointestinal tract, there is little evidence that any of the changes in gastrointestinal function (e.g. reduced gastric secretion, proximal gastric relaxation, small intestinal retroperistalsis) which occur in nauseated patients are actually the origin of the sensation via activation of visceral afferents [8]. More recent studies have demonstrated a relationship between nausea induced by illusory self-motion, pregnancy or unexplained causes and antral tachygastria, an increase in the frequency of gastric antral muscle electrical activity [41-44]. To date the only conclusion that can be drawn is that tachyantria often occurs in nauseated subjects but it is not the primary cause of the sensation, although the disturbed gastric motility associated with tachyantria could reinforce the sensation via vagal afferent activation.

Although the origin of the sensation of nausea has not yet been identified, studies in man are providing a much more accurate picture of the events occurring in nauseated subjects. Studies by Morrow et al. [5] have shown an increase in skin pallor, fall in skin temperature, decreased heart rate and blood volume pulse in patients with nausea receiving chemotherapy. Such studies used in combination with monitoring of endocrine changes (e.g. vasopressin, cortisol) and symptom questionnaires may provide the best approach to identifying the exact origin of the sensation.

Specific Mechanisms Involved in Triggering Anticancer Therapy-Induced Emesis

This section reviews the evidence from a number of preclinical studies in a variety of species for the mechanism by which anticancer therapies induce emesis. Although three phases of emesis (acute, delayed, anticipatory) have been described following various types of anticancer therapy, mechanistic studies have focussed on the acute phase as this is the most intense and is also the one most closely modelled in animal studies. Because of the nature of the types of study required to identify the pathways involved, we will probably never know exactly how closely the animal models resemble the situation in man. In addition, it is important to bear in mind that the experimental situation does not exactly mimic what happens in the clinic as the animals do not have a tumour burden, are not receiving concomitant medication (e.g. opiates) and have not had surgery (e.g. mastectomy). The psychological effects will also differ markedly between the experimental and clinical situations.

Because cisplatin is considered to evoke the most intense and prolonged emetic response in man, it has tended to be the focus for mechanistic studies, although the mechanisms identified appear to be used by a wide range of cytotoxic drugs and radiation. For an extensive review of the differences between the various animal models for cytotoxic and radiation-induced emesis the reader is referred to Andrews and Davis [4] and Harding et al. [45].

Acute

The acute phase of emesis is considered to be that which occurs immediately following administration of the cytotoxic drug or radiation. In man, for cisplatin the acute phase is considered to last 18-24 hours, although this definition is somewhat arbitrary [21,25,46-49]. The latency of onset differs relatively little, being between 1-2 hours in *Suncus*, ferret, cat, dog and monkey. Latencies between 1 and 6 hours are reported in man, depending upon the dose and rate of administration.

Although there are differences in the exact nature of the response to cisplatin, there is remarkable agreement across species in the mechanism by which this and other cytotoxic drugs induce emesis and these are reviewed in the next section.

Pathways by which Cytotoxic Drugs Induce Emesis

The original studies on the mechanism of both radiation and cytotoxic drug-induced emesis focussed on the role of the area postrema as at the time this was considered to be the detector of emetic agents in the circulation. Lesion studies of the area postrema showed variable results with complete protection being afforded against some agents in some species but with little effect being seen in other studies (see [4]). At the same time a few studies examined the effect of vagotomy either alone or in combination with greater splanchnic nerve section and showed that this lesion could also reduce emesis, again with inter-species and emetic agent differences. These differences were generally ascribed to differences in the degree to which each pathway was activated by the particular stimulus in each species. However, as more studies on the effect of abdominal visceral nerve lesions on the emetic response to a range of cytotoxic agents were undertaken in a number of species, it became clear that abdominal vagotomy was equivalent to area postrema ablation [4]. How can these apparently contradictory observations be reconciled? The explanation most consistent with the current evidence is that the primary site at which these cytotoxic agents and radiation act is in the gut wall to cause firing of the visceral afferents (predominantly vagus) which project to the brainstem. The main projection site for the abdominal vagal afferents is the superficial part of the nucleus tractus solitarius known as the subnucleus gelatinosus [19]. This site of termination is significant as it is immediately subjacent to the area postrema and hence the thermocautery lesions of the area postrema will inevitably cause some collateral damage to this region. In addition, there is evidence that some abdominal vagal afferents may actually terminate in the area postrema itself [19]. Thus lesion of the area postrema will interrupt the central projection of vagal afferent information to the emetic integrative and motor areas of the brainstem either indirectly (subnucleus gelatinosus lesion) or directly (area postrema ablation). Either explanation would account for the apparent equivalence of area postrema ablation and abdominal visceral nerve lesions against a range of cytotoxic drugs and radiation. Studies of brainstem neurone activation using the early immediate oncogene c-*fos* as a marker favour the first explanation because, although both the nucleus tractus solitarius and the area postrema have their activity increased by intravenous cisplatin in the ferret, it is only the activity in the former which is reduced by vagotomy which blocks the emetic response [50]. This study also demonstrates that cisplatin may have some direct effect on the area postrema and such an effect could include:

a) a facilitation of the emetic response to visceral or other stimuli with the area postrema modulating the sensitivity of the system;
b) effects on food and water intake functions in which the area postrema is known to have a role, particularly in the development of conditioned taste aversion;
c) the general behavioural changes associated with chemotherapy, e.g. lethargy.

The main problem with the above studies is that, although they cover a variety of species including a primate, we do not know which species most closely mimics man because it is not possible to undertake comparable studies in man. Bilateral abdominal vagotomy has been performed in man as a treatment for peptic ulcer but such surgery is now relatively uncommon with the advent of histamine$_2$ receptor antagonists (e.g. cimetidine) and proton pump inhibitors (e.g. omeprazole). In addition, when it is performed a more selective procedure is now used which only cuts the nerves supplying the proximal stomach. Thus the chances of studying a group of patients who have had a successful truncal vagotomy and who then go on to have a tumour (not involving the gut because of the direct emetic effects of obstruction) are low. It should also be remembered that in man vagotomy is usually accompanied by some additional gastric surgery such as pyloroplasty to facilitate gastric emptying and that nausea and vomiting are amongst the commonest side-effects of this operation. In addition, the "plasticity" of the emetic system reported in animal studies [51,26] will confound any such study because within a few weeks of the nerve lesion mechanisms not used when the vagus is present may be unmasked or induced. Patients with operable epidermoid cancer of the oesophagus will have vagotomy when the oesophagus is removed and an oesophagogastrostomy is performed [52]. Although this group would appear to be suitable for investigating the role of the vagus as chemotherapy and radiotherapy may be given both pre- and post-operatively, the extensive surgery to the gastrointestinal tract makes assessment of mechanisms impossible. Area postrema ablation has been used successfully in man to treat intractable vomiting [53] but this was a number of years ago and I am not aware of any more recent studies. In my opinion it is highly unlikely that ethical permission could be obtained to repeat this study, even if it were desirable, particularly in the light of our increased knowledge of the structure of the brainstem. In addition, even if such a study were undertaken in man, it would be open to the same problems of interpretation as the animal studies. At present the most convincing evidence that the mechanisms operating in man and the animal models are at least similar is the antiemetic efficacy of the 5-hydroxytryptamine$_3$ receptor antagonists in man and in a range of animal species.

Transformation of the Cytotoxic Stimulus into an Emetic Signal

If activation of the abdominal vagal afferents is the main route by which emesis is triggered by cytotoxic drugs and radiation, then the next question to ask is "How are the afferents activated?" The answer to this question has direct implications for identifying the best pharmacological approaches to blocking this activation. Two mechanisms must be considered: direct and indirect.

Direct

By this we mean that the cytotoxic drug or radiation interact directly with the afferent terminal in the gut wall (or area postrema neurones if this is considered a more likely site) to induce a neuronal discharge capable of inducing emesis. There are a number of pieces of evidence from studies of cisplatin which suggest that it may have some direct excitatory effects on neurones, although none of these have been directly linked to its emetic effects. Firstly, studies in the guinea-pig intestine have demonstrated an enteric cholinergic neural link in the pathway by which cisplatin induces the release of 5-HT from the mucosa [54]. Secondly, in the anaesthetised ferret cisplatin induces an immediate (<2 min latency) and transient (<15 min) stimulation of gastrointestinal motility which it was concluded was mediated by the release of acetylcholine from the myenteric nerves [55]. Thirdly, cisplatin in concentrations over the clinical range produced a dose-related (0.1-10 μM) decrease in the input conductance of cultured dorsal root ganglion neurones from neonatal rats [19]. These cells are the cell bodies of primary afferent neurones including those from the abdominal viscera, although not the vagal afferents. These conductance effects are indicative of an increased excitability and this is supported by a decrease in the threshold for activation of action potentials. Interestingly, the effects appeared to be stereospecific to a degree as transplatin was significantly less effective, an observation in accordance with the lack of antitumour effect of transplatin.

Although the above studies have revealed a novel mechanism by which cisplatin could act, this is probably not the major mechanism for the induction of emesis, although it is a likely candidate for facilitating the other mechanisms activated by cisplatin and may play a role in the emetic response in patients in which 5-HT$_3$ receptor antagonists have a reduced efficacy.

Indirect

Indirect activation of the emetic pathway could be brought about by the cytotoxic drug or radiation inducing the release of a substance capable of activating one or more of the emetic pathways. Because of the antiemetic efficacy of 5-HT$_3$ receptor antagonists against cytotoxic drugs including cisplatin, attention has focussed on understanding how and from where cisplatin could induce the release of 5-HT. The evidence for the involvement of 5-HT in emesis will only be outlined here as it has been the subject of recent extensive reviews [56,57]. A number of observations suggest that the gut is the most likely source of 5-HT:

a) The enterochromaffin cells (EC) in the mucosa of the gastrointestinal tract contain >80% of the 5-HT in the body;
b) abdominal visceral nerve lesions can markedly reduce or abolish the emetic response

to a variety of cytostatic stimuli (see above);

c) 5-HT_3 receptors are present on abdominal vagal afferents and activation of these afferents by 5-HT can be blocked by the 5-HT_3 receptor antagonists granisetron and ondansetron [58,59];

d) measurements of the levels of 5-HT in the mucosa of the intestine in ferrets treated with cisplatin showed that this agent altered the metabolism of 5-HT, leading to an increase in the levels in the ileal mucosa [57]. A marked increase in the release of 5-HT was induced by cisplatin in isolated ileal segments [60,61]. Although these and other studies provided a substantial circumstantial body of evidence for an involvement of the EC cell in cisplatin-induced emesis, it is only recently that the release of 5-HT has been directly measured in a species capable of vomiting [62], previous release studies having been performed in the guinea-pig. Using microdialysis, the change in the levels of 5-HT in the wall of the ileum were measured following cisplatin administration in the dog [62]. The level of 5-HT in the dialysate increased progressively after cisplatin, reaching a plateau between 100 and 180 min and declining to baseline levels by 280 min. Direct measurement of the level of 5-HT in the ileal mucosa removed 3 hours after cisplatin revealed an increased level, a finding consistent with earlier studies in the ferret. This observation is also consistent with the stimulation of 5-HT synthesis, which would be expected to accompany a markedly increased release from the EC cells. A study in the ferret reported that the increased release of 5-HT by cisplatin was accompanied by elevated activity of two synthetic enzymes, ileal tryptophan hydroxylase and aromatic-L-amino acid decarboxylase, and a decrease in monoamine oxidase [57]. Similar changes were also seen with cyclophosphamide and copper sulphate. The changes in these two enzymes will facilitate the increase in the local levels of 5-HT by enhancing the synthesis and reducing the degradation. Nausea and vomiting are typical side-effects of some mono-amine oxidase inhibitors and in the context of this chapter it is of interest that procarbazine was initially developed as an MAO inhibitor. The 5-HT released from the mucosa, if not metabolised to 5-hydroxy-indole acetic acid (5-HIAA) or taken back into the EC cells, would pass to the hepatic portal vein where it would be taken up into the platelets. Therefore, unless these mechanisms were saturated, an increase in the level of 5-HT in the plasma in the systemic circulation would not be expected. In man, studies in patients receiving cisplatin have shown an increase in the plasma and urine concentrations of 5-HIAA with a time course corresponding to the pattern of acute emesis. In general, there has been little evidence that systemic blood levels (either in the plasma or in erythrocytes, [63]) of 5-HT increase following cytotoxic drugs, although one study [64] reported a transient but marked (500 to 1000%) increase in 4 out of 10 patients; however, the times at which the levels peaked were variable (4 hrs and 8 hrs). In the dog it was found that, in contrast to the ileal levels which began to increase immediately after the cisplatin, plasma levels did not appear to increase until after the animal had begun vomiting (~2hrs), and returned to basal levels at 240 mins, when emesis stopped [62]. Because of the temporal dissociation between the rise in plasma 5-HT and the onset of emesis it is unlikely that it is the 5-HT level in the plasma that is responsible for triggering emesis by an action at a site such as the area postrema. A more likely explanation is that the increase in 5-HT is due to mechanical stimulation of the intestines by vomiting, inducing a release of 5-HT from the mucosa which adds to the cisplatin-induced 5-HT release resulting in swamping of the platelet uptake mechanism leading to an increase in the plasma levels. Interestingly, the release of 5-HT by the mechanical stimulus of vomiting could provide a positive feedback to optimise the expulsive response when the system is challenged.

To summarise, the vast weight of evidence from release and histological studies favours the enterochromaffin cells of the small intestine as the site from which 5-HT is released by the action of cytotoxic drugs and radiation. The mechanism by which the 5-HT is released is not fully understood but the generation of free radicals appears to be an intermediate step as experiments in the insectivore *Suncus murinus* have shown that emesis induced by the free radical generator pyrogallol can be blocked by a 5-HT_3 receptor antagonist (tropisetron). It was also demonstrated that the emetic response to cisplatin was blocked by the antioxidant N-(2-mercaptoproprionyl)-glycine [65, 66]. Recent studies in the guinea-pig suggest that the release of 5-HT is under the control of 5-HT autoreceptors located on the EC cells [66]. It is proposed that a 5-HT_4 receptor sensitive to "low" concentrations of 5-HT provides an inhibitory negative feedback to 5-HT release under physiological conditions. Blower and Andrews [unpublished] have proposed that when the release of 5-HT is "high" under pathophysiological conditions (e.g. induced by cisplatin or radiation), a 5-HT_3 receptor also located on the EC cell becomes activated and provides a positive feedback to 5-HT release which cannot be offset by the limited inhibition produced by the 5-HT_4 receptor. This positive feedback would provide a means of rapidly amplifying the emetic signal to produce a prompt and intense emetic response. The 5-HT released appears to have a predominantly local action to activate 5-HT_3 receptors located on vagal afferents terminating in close proximity. Although 5-HT is the focus of attention, it should be borne in mind that other neuroactive agents (e.g. Substance P, noradrenaline, CCK) may also be released from the intestinal mucosa and potentiate the response to 5-HT.

Although the studies on the release of 5-HT provide the most direct evidence for its involvement in emesis, indirect supportive evidence comes from studies of the dose of 5-HT_3 receptor antagonist required to block emesis and two studies illustrate this approach. Using two doses of total body radiation in the ferret it was demonstrated that a higher dose of granisetron was required to reduce emesis by 50% at the higher dose of radiation than the lower [26]. The emetic response to both doses could be blocked by this agent if the dose of antagonist was sufficiently high. In man, a comparison was made of the efficacy of a fixed dose of ondansetron against highly (cisplatin) and moderately (cyclophosphamide-based combination) emetic cytotoxic regimes. A higher complete response rate was found in the group receiving the moderately emetic regime. Both studies support the hypothesis that proportional release of 5-HT and degree of activation of 5-HT_3 receptors are the link between the cytostatic treatment and emesis.

Possible Mechanisms Involved in Delayed Emesis

With cytotoxic drugs such as cisplatin, carboplatin and cyclophosphamide the nausea and vomiting may continue for several days after an initial intense acute phase in the first 18-24 hours. The exact point at which the acute phase ends and the delayed phase begins is at present somewhat arbitrary but this may improve as the mechanism underlying the phases becomes apparent. Studies with the 5-HT_3 receptor antagonists have already provided some insights into this problem. Typically, the 5-HT_3 receptor antagonists (granisetron [Kytril], ondansetron [Zofran], tropisetron [Navoban]) have their major antiemetic effects in the first 18-24 hours [67-69], indicating that the predominant mechanism in the acute phase is as outlined in the section above. Outside this period the involvement of 5-HT_3 receptors appears to be small, although it is important to bear in mind that this does not exclude an involvement for 5-HT acting on another receptor type. Studies by Cubeddu et al. [70] have shown that urine 5-HIAA levels remain elevated above control levels (although not statistically significant) up to 4 days after cisplatin, although they gradually declined after the first 24 hours. It is possible that in this phase the 5-HT is more active in sensitising the emetic system rather than driving it, as in the acute phase. A number of animal studies have shown long-lasting structural changes induced by cytotoxic drugs but similar detailed studies have not been undertaken in man. Studies in the dog have shown an increase in the number of 5-HT immunoreactive cells in the ileum 3 hours after cisplatin administration [62] and histopathological changes including karyohexis are seen at 6 hours in the ferret [60]. In ferrets given two doses of cisplatin 24 hours apart and examined 3 hours after the second dose, congestion of the lamina propria is seen accompanied by glandular necrosis and some haemorrhage [60, 61]. In the mouse, cisplatin reduced villus height starting 3 days after injection and lasting up to 10 days, accompanied by a reduction in sucrase and maltase. Crypt cell production was also severely reduced and the normal cell dynamics of the crypt and villus only began to be restored between 5 and 7 days [71,72]. The functional impact of these structural changes is likely to be extensive and some of the possibilities are outlined below.

They could be accompanied by increased permeability of the mucosa, allowing endotoxin lipopolysaccharides (LPS) into the bloodstream. These are derived from bacteria such as *E. Coli* and when given intravenously are known to induce emesis. In man, a dramatic rise in plasma LPS reaching a peak over 4 days has been reported in patients undergoing radiotherapy of the cervix [73]. The LPS levels were related to the morbidity index. In addition, damage to the intestinal mucosa has been implicated in the mechanism by which viral infections may cause prolonged disruption of gastrointestinal motility which could contribute an emetic signal. In the rat and mouse, single doses of cisplatin produce a dose-related inhibition of gastric emptying which may last several days, approximately mimicking the time course of delayed emesis [74]. From this brief outline it appears likely that some degree of disruption of upper gastrointestinal function is involved in delayed emesis and this observation is to some extent supported by the beneficial effect of conventional doses of prokinetic drugs such as metoclopramide and alizapride in delayed emesis. It is worth cautioning that with the introduction of 5-HT_3 receptor antagonists many patients now feel like taking food in the first 24 hours after chemotherapy. If, as is suspected, gastrointestinal tract function is disrupted for several days, patients should be given some dietary advice to avoid large meals, fatty food and hypertonic drinks, all of which slow gastric emptying and can be emetic in healthy subjects.

The corticosteroid analogue dexamethasone and related steroids (e.g. methylprednisolone) are used in the treatment of delayed emesis but their mechanism of action in this and the acute phase is not known, although proposed mechanisms mostly based on studies of non-emetic mechanisms include: reduction of a low-grade cerebral oedema induced by cytotoxic drugs, tightening of capillaries in the brain or gut to limit access of toxins which may stimulate emetic pathways, general anti-inflammatory effects reducing damage to the gut mucosa, modulation of receptor regulation or intracellular messenger systems (e.g. Ca^{++}), reduction of 5-HT turnover in the central nervous system and stabilisation of neurones in the emetic pathways to reduce their excitability to emetic stimuli. In man, no evidence has been found that dexamethasone reduces the release of 5-HT (as indicated by urinary 5-HIAA) induced by high-dose cisplatin in the acute phase of emesis [63].

Support for the involvement of endogenous steroids in delayed emesis comes from a study in a variety of chemotherapy patients showing that subjects with high night-time urinary cortisol excretion prior to treatment had a lower nausea score for the first two days after treatment [75]. Circulating noradrenaline may also be involved as pretreatment nocturnal plasma noradrenaline levels predicted the incidence and intensity of nausea in the delayed phase [76].

It will be apparent from the above discussion that there is very little hard information about the precise mechanisms underlying the delayed phase of emesis, although the general impression is that it is likely to be multi-factorial, with the predominant mechanism altering with time. Whilst the efficacy of mild prokinetic agents can be rationalised, there is no equivalent satisfactory explanation for dexamethasone, although its obvious efficacy in delayed emesis gives a clear pointer that its mechanism of action is worthy of study. The identification of the mechanism of delayed emesis has been hampered by the lack of an animal model, but a recent report in the ferret suggests that a lower dose (5 mg/kg, i.p.) of cisplatin than normally used (10 mg/kg, i.p.) may induce a long-lasting (3 days) emetic response with many features of delayed emesis in man [76]. Whilst 5-HT_3 receptor antagonists reduced the emetic response on days 2 and 3, they did not block it, thus supporting the contention that this model may be of use in identifying the mechanisms involved in man [77]. In contrast, the neurokinin$_1$ receptor antagonist CP-99,994 had a profound inhibitory effect on both the acute and delayed phase of emesis induced by cisplatin in the ferret [78,79]. A piglet model for the study of the delayed phase of emesis induced by cisplatin has recently been described [80].

In contrast to the studies in man and the ferret, this piglet study implicates 5-HT and 5-HT_3 receptors in the delayed phase [80]. It is clear that further human and animal studies need to be undertaken before the mechanism(s) of delayed emesis and the underlying pharmacology can be understood.

Interactions Between Acute and Delayed Phases

The studies with 5-HT_3 receptor antagonists indicate that the two phases are not causally linked as blockade of the acute phase does not mean that a delayed phase will not occur. Because the delayed phase has been so poorly quantified it is impossible to say whether blockade of the acute phase modifies the delayed phase. However, this would not be surprising if only from the aspect that, if the patient has not vomited in the acute phase, he will less expect to vomit with increasing time from therapy. Further studies in man are needed to identify the interactions between the two phases.

One possible interaction between the acute and delayed phases which may become apparent relates to the blockade of emesis in the acute phase by 5-HT_3 receptor antagonists. Patients who do not experience emesis in the acute phase after cytotoxic treatment are likely to feel sufficiently well to want food and such an effect has been observed in a study with ondansetron [77]. However, their gastrointestinal tract function (motility and transport) will still be disturbed by the cytotoxic drug and particularly cisplatin. Thus a functionally compromised gut is expected to deal with a meal in the normal way. It is therefore possible that some of the delayed emesis seen in patients protected during the first 24 hours is contributed to by this disturbed gastrointestinal function. It may become necessary to give patients dietary advice to reduce any such effect.

Anticipatory Nausea and Vomiting

Anticipatory nausea and vomiting (ANV) is that occurring prior to treatment. Although ANV may rarely occur before the first course of therapy because of the patient's expectation (often unjustified) of the unpleasant nature of the experience, it is more common once therapy has started. Studies by Morrow et al. [5] have shown that the incidence relates to the number of courses of therapy and the degree of antiemetic control, although the mechanisms underlying individual susceptibility to ANV are not known. The most widely accepted mechanism for the induction of ANV is that it represents an example of Pavlovian classical conditioning [2]. In this model the chemotherapy is the unconditioned stimulus and nausea and vomiting are the unconditioned responses. However, a learned association may be made between a variety of aspects of the chemotherapy (the conditioned stimuli) and the nausea and vomiting. Such stimuli can be the sight of the chemotherapy nurse or the hospital, the smell of the ward or the taste associated with some cytotoxic drugs. Thus nausea and vomiting can eventually be induced by one of these stimuli or indeed even by the thought of them. It appears likely that the fundamental biological process of classical conditioning or associative learning will be modified by the patient's previous emetic history and also by the psychological impact of cancer and chemotherapy.

It is important to reiterate that the generation of an aversive response to a cytotoxic drug is an appropriate biological response and is a component of the body's defensive system against accidentally ingested toxins. The central nervous system pathways involved in such responses are not known but the phenomenon of "conditioned taste aversion" in animals which involves the area postrema shares some similarities with ANV, although it is by no means equivalent [81].

It can be argued that the best way to "treat" ANV is to prevent its development by developing totally effective antiemetics so that neither acute nor delayed emesis will occur in response to any type of anticancer therapy. The introduction of the 5-HT_3 receptor antagonists has gone some way to achieving this in many patients and it will be interesting to assess their impact on ANV. Even if universally active antiemetics are developed it is likely that some patients may still experience some nausea from purely psychological factors because they expect to experience nausea when undergoing chemotherapy. For this reason it is important that developments in antiemetic therapy are paralleled by patient education programmes so that new patients gain an accurate picture of the experience of anticancer therapy rather than one based on out-of-date anecdote and hearsay.

Once ANV has developed it is very difficult to treat. Psychological techniques such as hypnosis, relaxation training and systematic desensitisation are the most useful, especially if used prior to therapy [2,3,5]. As ANV relies on the development of an associative memory, drugs with an amnesic and sedative action such as the benzodiazepines have been found to be useful.

Is the Mechanism of Emesis in the First and Subsequent Cycles the Same?

The answer to this question is probably 'yes', although some qualification is required. Studies in the ferret giving emetic doses of cisplatin on consecutive days show that in general the response on the second day is better, but whether this is due to accumulation of cisplatin or sensitisation of the emetic system is unclear. In addition, the emetic response on the second day could be blocked by an adequate dose of a 5-HT_3 receptor antagonist, as is the case with the response following a single dose of cisplatin, i.e., suggesting that the same mechanism is involved. This study parallels the situation in fractionated chemotherapy where granisetron has been shown to be effective over 5 days of therapy with cisplatin, ifosfamide or etoposide [82].

In man, Cubeddu et al. [70,83] have shown similar increases in urinary 5-HIAA on the first and up to 4 subsequent courses of cisplatin treatment. The efficacy of 5-HT_3 receptor antagonists over multiple cycles of therapy supports the contention that 5-HT has a major involvement in the first and subsequent cycles, although there appears to be a general trend towards a reduction in the overall efficacy with increasing numbers of cycles. This reduction appears to be more pronounced in female patients [82]. One explanation for these observations is that additional non-5-HT_3 emetic mechanisms are being recruited. These could include an increasing drive from higher centres due to psychological factors or recruitment of other mechanisms such as the release of emetic peptides from the gut, as has been suggested to be involved in the emetic response to high-dose radiation in the absence of the vagus. Further studies are needed in man to carefully document the nature of the emetic response (e.g. latency, magnitude, duration) in patients undergoing multiple cycles of highly emetic chemotherapy therapy. In addition, it is important to examine the response of individual patients in order to see whether patients with a poor response on the first cycle continue to respond poorly or whether good responders progressively deteriorate.

Is There a Physiological Basis for Predisposing and Protecting Factors?

A number of prognostic factors have been identified for chemotherapy-induced emesis and provide a useful guide to identifying the patients who may be most at risk. Whilst the physiological and pharmacological basis for the intensity of emesis induced by the various agents is clear (as is the efficacy of the various antiemetics), the mechanisms underlying some of the other factors have seldom been discussed. Although the factors are discussed in isolation, they will interact in a complex manner in an individual patient and this is illustrated by the increase in their utility as prognostic factors when they are examined in combination (e.g. see statistical analysis by Morrow [3]). Psychological predisposing factors have been reviewed recently by Cull [2] and Andryowski [84] and will not be discussed here.

Emetic History and Motion Sensitivity

From our understanding of the mechanism of anticipatory nausea and vomiting to chemotherapy it is easy to appreciate that poor emetic control on the first cycle can increase the probability of emesis during subsequent cycles. Less attention has been focussed on the effect of previous emetic experience from non-therapeutic causes. Motion is probably the most common emetic stimulus to which the general population is exposed and there appears to be a positive relationship between motion sensitivity and the probability of development of anticipatory emesis [85]. It is unclear whether the sensitivity to motion sickness and chemotherapy agents are both indicators of a sensitive emetic system in these patients or whether the emetic system has become sensitised over the years by repeated exposure to an emetic stimulus. It would be of interest to know the predictive value of other emetic stimuli such as food poisoning and migraine. Identifying the mechanisms underlying these relationships is confounded by the influence of age and gender which are outlined below.

Age and Gender

Most data on the influence of age and gender on emetic sensitivity come from studies of motion sickness. Infants below the age of two are considered to be immune to motion sickness but sensitivity soon rises, with the highest level incidence between 2 and 12 years. Above this age the incidence falls and appears to continue to fall throughout adult life, with any form of motion sickness being reported to be very rare above the age of 50 [86]. The incidence of postoperative nausea and vomiting (PONV) increases until puberty and in general appears to decline with age. It is more commonly encountered in females than males [87,88]. The exact incidence of PONV is multi-factorial, depending, for example, upon type of anaesthetic, surgery, and concomitant medication. The mechanism of PONV is not known [89].

The extent to which age is a prognostic factor in acute cytotoxic emesis is still a matter of debate. Anecdotally the young (~<16 yrs) are considered to be more susceptible. It is also assumed that the elderly (90) are less susceptible but this is not a universal finding. Age under 50 years is considered to be one of the 8 prognostic factors for predicting susceptibility to anticipatory nausea and vomiting [91].

A further indication that "older" age may be protective comes from studies of the effect of age on the efficacy of antiemetics. Emesis is better controlled in patients older than 50 years by a 5-HT_3 receptor antagonist (tropisetron) than in young adults [67]. For example, in a study of children between 2 and 16 years undergoing various types of chemotherapy, tropisetron had a complete response rate of 69% in the acute phase [67], illustrating that in both children and adults the predominant mechanism of cytotoxic emesis involves 5-HT_3 receptor activation. This contention is confirmed by the observation that granisetron reduced or abolished radiation or cyclophosphamide + doxorubicin-induced emesis in juvenile as well as adult ferrets [92].

Women have a higher incidence of motion sickness than men and have a tendency to adapt more slowly to repetitive nauseogenic stimuli [92]. If this reduced rate of adaptation can be generalised then it could go some way towards explaining the reduced efficacy of 5-HT_3 receptor antagonists in women compared to men undergoing multiple cycles of chemotherapy (see above). Some studies report that motion sensitivity is higher during menstruation, which is consistent with reports of an increased incidence of postoperative nausea and vomiting during menstruation [94].

These differences in motion sensitivity appear to apply to chemotherapy, even when allowances are made for the different types of therapy and cancer site as women experience a higher rate of nausea and vomiting than males. In addition, the intensity of nausea, number of vomiting episodes and duration of nausea and vomiting are greater in females [95]. The incidence of delayed emesis is also reported to be higher in women than in men. Emetic experience during previous pregnancy has also been reported to modify the emetic response to the FAC regime (doxorubicin, 5-FU, cyclophosphamide) [96]. Protection from emesis was only found in 36% of women in whom emesis was present for the whole day during the first trimester or extended beyond, in contrast to complete protection in 85% of women who had experienced no pregnancy sickness.

The mechanism underlying these sex differences is unclear and has not been the subject of basic studies but the most plausible hypothesis is that the female sex steroids sensitise the central emetic pathways so that the response to many types of emetic input is heightened. A similar hypothesis has been proposed to account for the induction of pregnancy sickness [97] and is supported by the observation that emesis can be induced by oestrogen therapy. Preliminary studies by Cubeddu et al. [70] failed to demonstrate a difference between men and women in the amount of 5-HT released in response to high-dose cisplatin, supporting the hypothesis that it is the sensitivity of the emetic pathways that differs rather than the driving stimulus. In the context of antiemetic therapy it is of interest that the steroid dexamethasone appears to have a more beneficial effect on females than males when used in combination with a 5-HT_3 receptor antagonist (granisetron).

Alcohol

It has been reported that a high level (>100 g/day) of chronic alcohol consumption markedly reduced or completely abolished the emetic effects of cisplatin, although this is not a universal finding and requires further investigation [98]. Whilst damage to central nervous system structures involved in the emetic response would seem an obvious mechanism and one consistent with the known effects of chronic ethanol consumption, a possible effect on abdominal visceral afferents (an alcoholic autonomic neuropathy) or enterochromaffin cells should not be overlooked.

Race

Possible racial differences in emetic sensitivity have not been investigated for cytotoxic emesis but studies of motion sensitivity indicate that such differences may exist. Using vection (illusory self-motion) as the stimulus, Chinese subjects were shown to have significantly increased nausea responses when compared with Caucasian and African-American subjects [101]. Preliminary studies suggest that the vasopressin release related to nausea was greater in Chinese than Caucasian subjects [102]. Studies of racial (and cultural) differences in emetic sensitivity to cytotoxic therapy may give insight into basic emetic mechanisms and assist our understanding of differences seen in multi-national clinical trials.

The Future

The past 10 years have seen considerable advances in our understanding of emetic mechanisms. However, there are a number of outstanding issues which require investigation before it can be said that the problem of emesis associated with cytotoxic therapy has been solved. Some of these mechanistic issues are outlined below.

Translation of Animal Studies to Man

Whilst studies in appropriate animal models can clearly demonstrate the antiemetic efficacy of a novel drug, it is often found that the drug is less efficacious in man. In contrast to patients receiving cytotoxic drugs, the animals do not have a tumour burden, are not receiving concomitant medication and are not exposed to the same psychological influences. Further consideration should be given to the way in which these factors can modify the sensitivity of the emetic reflex and how they interact with the better defined prognostic factors (see above).

Although animal studies have provided much of our understanding of the physiology and pharmacology of the emetic reflex in general, far fewer studies have investigated the reflex directly in man. Because of this relative paucity of information it is sometimes difficult to assess how close the animal models come to the situation in man. This is a particular problem when trying to identify the neural pathways used by the various emetic stimuli. However, parallel pharmacological studies in man and animals with the 5-HT_3 receptor antagonists and, more recently, using the 5-HT synthesis inhibitor para-chlorophenylalanine [103], have shown considerable general similarities in the involvement of 5-HT in emesis in man and animals. It is hoped that similar parallels will apply to the involvement of NK-1 receptors [78,79].

A further difficulty with extrapolating the results from animal studies to man concerns nausea. In animals it is only possible to measure the "behavioural correlates" of nausea rather than the reported subjective sensation itself, which is possible in man. It is essential that reliable objective physiological markers (e.g. tachygastria, plasma vasopressin) are identified for nausea in man which can be applied to animal studies. At present it is conceivable that animal studies could identify an agent which completely blocks retching and vomiting but which, when studied in man, has no effect on nausea, although completely blocking mechanical components of the emetic reflex.

The Requirement for Novel Antiemetics

Because it is not possible to block all components of the emetic response in all patients treated with cytotoxic drugs or radiation, there is a clear requirement for novel antiemetic agents. Studies in animals have provided a strong indication that $neurokinin_1$ receptor antagonists may be more general antiemetics than 5-HT_3

receptor antagonists and therefore be capable of blocking both acute and delayed emesis [78,79]. Studies in patients of this class of agent are eagerly awaited. In addition to neurokinin$_1$ receptor antagonists, other approaches under investigation include excitatory amino-acid receptor antagonists [104] and agents with mixed actions acting as agonists on 5-HT$_1$ receptors and antagonists on 5-HT$_3$ receptors [105].

Cellular Effects of Cisplatin and Dexamethasone

Studies of the cellular effects of cisplatin and other cytotoxic drugs have focussed on toxicity [106] and in general have not attempted to identify more pharmacological effects. The identification of the enterochromaffin cell as a major target for the emetic effects of cytotoxic drugs has stimulated interest in the cellular effects. The electrophysiological effects of acute and chronic (5-7 days) exposure of cultured dorsal root ganglion cells to cisplatin (5 μM) have been investigated [19,107]. Acutely, cisplatin decreased the input resistance and transiently increased cell excitability. Chronic application markedly reduced voltage-activated potassium currents and calcium currents but the inward cation current activated by hyperpolarisation was doubled. It appears that cisplatin perturbs calcium homeostatic mechanism in these cells. Such an action has been reported to contribute to cisplatin toxicity in other systems [106]. Although the antiemetic effects of dexamethasone are well established [e.g. 108], the mechanism of action is not known. This problem has been approached using the cultured dorsal root ganglion to characterise the electrophysiological effects of dexamethasone and its interaction with cisplatin [107]. Acute application of dexamethasone (1-10 μM) produced transient depolarisation and bursts of action potentials but by 5 min after application there was no effect on membrane potential, input resistance or evoked action potentials. An observation of potential clinical relevance was that dexamethasone improved the survival (20% increase) and electrophysiological properties of cells exposed chronically to 5 μM cisplatin. The mechanism of this "neuroprotective" effect is not known but a similar effect has been reported using a functional assay (5-HT-induced depolarisation) in rat cervical vagal axons [109]. This effect, if it can be demonstrated *in vivo*, is of particular interest as dexamethasone does not protect tumour cells from the effects of cisplatin [110]. The mechanism of this action of dexamethasone and its relationship (if any) to its antiemetic effects is unclear but both may relate to the reduction in free radical generation which can be produced by dexamethasone [111].

It is anticipated that answers to the above problems will be forthcoming in the next 5 years and will, hopefully, provide as dramatic an advance in our understanding of cytotoxic drug and radiation-induced emesis as have the 5-HT$_3$ receptor antagonists. Attention can then focus on finding treatment for other adverse effects of therapy, such as fatigue and weakness, which markedly reduce oncology patients' quality of life.

REFERENCES

1 Andrews PLR: Vomiting: a gastrointestinal tract defensive reflex. In: Andrews PLR and Widdicombe JG (eds) Pathophysiology of the Gut and Airways. Portland Press, London, UK 1993 pp 97-11

2 Cull A: Psychological effects of anti-cancer therapy: In: Andrews PLR and Sanger GJ: Emesis in Anti-Cancer Therapy, Mechanisms and Treatment. Chapman and Hall Medical, London 1993 pp 211-228

3 Morrow GR: Behavioural factors influencing the development and expression of chemotherapy induced side effects. Br J Cancer 1992 (66 Suppl 14):S54-S61

4 Andrews PLR and Davis CJ: The mechanism of emesis induced by anti-cancer therapies. In: Andrews PLR and Sanger GJ (eds) Emesis in Anti-Cancer Therapy, Mechanisms and Treatment. Chapman and Hall Medical, London 1993 pp 113-162

5 Morrow GR, Angel C, Dubeshter B: Autonomic changes during cancer chemotherapy induced nausea and emesis. Br J Cancer 1992 (66 Suppl XIX): S42-45

6 Lang IM: New perspectives on the mechanism controlling vomitus expulsion. In: Bianchi AL, Grelot L, Miller AD, King GL (eds) Mechanisms and Control of Emesis. Colloque INSERM, John Libbey, Eurotext 1993 (223):71-80

7 De Ponti F, Malagelada J, Azpiroz F, Yaksh TL, Thomforde GM: Variations in gastric tone associated with duodenal motor events after activation of central emetic mechanisms in the dog. J Gastrointestinal Motility 1990 (2):1-11

8 Lang IM: Digestive tract motor correlates of nausea and vomiting. Can J Physiol Pharmacol 1990 (68): 242-253

9 Monges H, Salducci J, Naudy B: Dissociation between the electrical activity of the diaphragmatic dome and crura muscular fibres during oesophageal distention, vomiting and eructation. An electromyographic study in the dog. J Physiol (Paris) 1978 (74):541-554

10 Koga T and Fukuda H: Characteristic behaviour of the respiratory muscles, esophagus, and external anal and urethral sphincters during straining, retching and vomiting in the decerebrate dog. Jap J Physiol 1990 (40):789-807

11 Andrews PLR, Bhandari P, Garland et al: Does retching have a function? An experimental study in the ferret. Pharmacodyn Ther (Life Sci Adv) 1990 (9):135-152

12 Miller AD, Nonaka S, Jakus J: Brain areas essential or non-essential for emesis. Brain Res 1994 (647): 255-264

13 Koga T and Fukuda H: Neurons in the nucleus of the solitary tract mediating inputs from emetic vagal afferents and the area postrema to the pattern generator for the emetic act in dogs. Neurosci Res 1992 (14):166-179

14 Mehler WR: Observations on the connectivity of the parvicellular reticular formation with respect to the vomiting centre. Brain Behav Evol 1983 (23): 63-80

15 Fukuda H and Koga T: The Bötzinger complex as the pattern generator for retching and vomiting in the dog. Neurosci Res 1991 (12):471-485

16 Fukuda H and Koga T: Non-respiratory neurons in the Bötzinger complex exhibiting appropriate firing patterns to generate the emetic act in dogs. Neurosci Res 1992 (14):180-194

17 Costello DJ and Borison HL: Naloxone antagonises narcotic self-blockade of emesis in the cat. J Pharmacol Exp Ther 1977 (203):222-230

18 Borison HL: Area postrema: Chemoreceptor circumventricular organ of the medulla oblongata. Prog Neurobiol 1989 (32):351-390

19 Scott R, Manikon MI, Andrews PLR: Actions of cisplatin on the electrophysiological properties of cultured dorsal root ganglion neurones from neonatal rats. Naunyn-Schmiedeberg's Arch Pharmacol 1994 (349):287-294

20 Harris AL: Cytotoxic therapy induced vomiting is mediated via enkephalin pathways. Lancet 1982 (1):714-716

21 Matsuki N, Torii Y, Ueno S, Saito H: Suncus murinus as an experimental animal model for emesis and motion sickness. In: Bianchi AL, Grelot L, Miller AD, King GL (eds) Mechanisms and Control of Emesis. Colloque INSERM, J Libbey, Eurotext 1992 (223):323-329

22 Herrstedt J, Hytetel J, Pedersen J: Interaction of the anti-emetic metopimozine and anti-cancer agents with brain dopamine D2, 5-hydroxytryptamine3, histamine1, muscarinic cholinergic and alpha-1 adrenergic receptors. Cancer Chemother Pharmacol 1993 (33):53-56

23 Carpenter DO, Briggs DB, Knox AP, Strominger N: Excitation of area postrema neurons by transmitters, peptides and cyclic nucleotides. J Neurophysiol 1988 (59):358-369

24 Grundy DG and Scratcherd T: Sensory afferents from the gastrointestinal tract. In: Wood JD (ed) Handbook of Physiology, Section 6, Vol 1, Part 1. American Physiological Society, Bethesda, Maryland, USA 1989 pp 593-620

25 Hawthorn J, Ostler KJ, Andrews PLR: The role of the abdominal visceral innervation and 5-hydroxytryptamine-M receptors in vomiting induced by the cytotoxic drugs cyclophosphamide and cisplatin in the ferret. Q J Exp Physiol 1988 (73):7-21

26 Andrews PLR, Bhandari P, Davis CJ: Plasticity and modulation of the emetic reflex. In: Bianchi AL, Grelot L, Miller AD, King GL (eds) Mechanisms and Control of Emesis. Colloque INSERM, John Libbey, Eurotext 1992 (223):275-284

27 Isaacs B: The influence of head and body position on the emetic action of apomorphine in man. Clin Science 1957 (16):215-221

28 Sem-Jacobsen CW: Depth Electrographic Stimulation of the Human Brain and Behaviour. Thomas, Springfield, IIL 1968

29 Robinson BW and Mishkin M: Alimentary responses to forebrain stimulation in monkeys. Exp Brain Res 1968 (4):330-366

30 Fennegan FM and Puiggari MJ: Hypothalamic and amygdaloid influence on gastric motility in dogs. J Neurosurg 1966 (24):497-504

31 Muraoka M, Mine K, Matsumoto K, Nakai Y, Nakagawa T: Psychogenic vomiting: the relation between patterns of vomiting and psychiatric diagnosis. Gut 1990 (31):526-528

32 Borison HL, Brand ED, Orkland RK: Emetic action of nitrogen mustard (mechlorethamine hydrochloride) in dogs and cats. Am J Physiol 1958 (192):410-416

33 Koch KL, Summy-Long J, Bingaman S, Sperry N, Stern RM: Vasopressin and oxytocin responses to illusory self-motion and nausea in man. J Clin Endocrinol Metab 1990 (71):1269-1275

34 Feldman M, Samson WK, O'Dorisio TM: Apomorphine-induced nausea in humans: release of vasopressin and pancreatic polypeptide. Gastroenterology 1988 (95):721-726

35 Nussey SS, Hawthorn J, Page SR, Ang VTY, Jenkins JS: Responses of plasma oxytocin and arginine vasopressin to nausea induced by apomorphine and ipecacuanha. Clin Endocrinol 1988 (28):297-304

36 Edwards CM, Carmichael J, Baylis PH, Harris AL: Arginine vasopressin - a mediator of chemotherapy-induced emesis? Br J Cancer 1989 (59):467-470

37 Hawthorn J, Andrews PLR, Ang VTY, Jenkins JS: Differential release of vasopressin and oxytocin in response to abdominal vagal afferent stimulation or apomorphine in the ferret. Brain Research 1988 (438):193-198

38 Verbalis JG, Richardson DW, Stricker EM: Vasopressin release in response to nausea producing agents and cholecystokinin in monkeys. Am J Physiol 1987 (252):R749-753

39 Thomford NR and Sirinek KR: Intravenous vasopressin in patients with portal hypertension. J Surg Res 1975 (18):113-117

40 Kohl RL and MacDonald S: New pharmacologic approaches to the prevention of space/motion sickness. J Clin Pharmacol 1991 (31):934-946

41 Clevers GH, Smout AJPM, Van Der Schee EJ, Akkermans LM: Changes in gastric electrical activity in patients with severe postoperative nausea and vomiting. J Gastrointest Mot 1992 (4):61-69

42 Stern RM, Koch KL, Stewart WR, Lindblad IM: Spectral analysis of tachygastria recorded during motion sickness. Gastroenterology 1987 (92):92-97

43 Geldof H, van der Schee EJ, van Blankenstein M, Grashuis JL: Electrogastrographic study of gastric myoelectrical activity in patients with unexplained nausea and vomiting. Gut 1986 (27):799-808

44 Xu LH, Koch KL, Summy-Long J et al: Hypothalamic and gastric myoelectrical response during vection-induced nausea in healthy Chinese subjects. Am J Physiol 1993 (265):E578-584

45 Harding RK, Young RW, Anno GH: Radiotherapy-induced emesis. In: Andrews PLR and Sanger GJ (eds) Emesis in Anti-Cancer Therapy: Mechanisms and Treatment. Chapman and Hall Medical, London 1993 pp 163-178

46 McCarthy LE and Borison HL: Cisplatin-induced vomiting eliminated by ablation of the area postrema in cats. Cancer Treat Rep 1984 (68):401-404

47 Fukui H, Yamamoto M, Sasaki S, Sato S: Emetic effects of anticancer drugs and involvement of visceral afferent fibres and 5-HT3 receptors in dogs. Eur J Pharmacol 1993 (250):281-287

48 Fukui H, Yamamoto M, Sato S: Vagal afferent fibres and peripheral 5-HT3 receptors mediate cisplatin-induced emesis in dogs. Jap J Pharmacol 1992 (59):221-222

49 Fukui HM, Yamamoto S, Sasaki S, Sato S: Involvement of 5-HT3 receptors and vagal afferents in copper sulphate and cisplatin-induced emesis in monkeys. Eur J Pharmacol 1993 (249):13-18

50 Reynolds DJM, Barber NA, Grahame-Smith DG, Leslie RA: Cisplatin-evoked induction of c-fos protein in the brainstem of the ferret: the effect of cervical vagotomy and the anti-emetic 5-HT3 receptor antagonist granisetron (BRL 43694). Brain Res 1991 (565):231-236

51 Andrews PLR, Davis CJ, Bingham S, Davidson HIM, Hawthorn J, Maskell L: The abdominal visceral innervation and the emetic reflex: pathways, pharmacology and plasticity. Can J Physiol Pharmacol 1990 (68):325-345

52 Kelsen DP, Minsky B, Smith M, Beitler J, Niedzwiecki D, Chapman D, Bains M, Burt M, Heelan R, Hilaris B: Preoperative therapy for oesophageal cancer: A randomized comparison of chemotherapy versus radiation therapy. J Clin Oncol 1990 (8): 1352-1361

53 Lindstrom PA and Brizzee KR: Relief of intractable vomiting from surgical lesions in the area postrema. J Neurosurg 1962 (19):228-236

54 Schwörer H, Racke K, Kilbinger H: Cisplatin increases the release of 5-hydroxytryptamine (5-HT) from the isolated vascularly perfused small intestine of the guinea pig: Involvement of 5-HT3 receptors. Naunyn-Schmiedeberg's Arch Pharmacol 1991 (344):143-149

55 Davidson HIM and Andrews PLR: Stimulation of gastrointestinal motility by cisplatin in the ferret: activation of an intrinsic cholinergic mechanism dissociated from emesis. Naunyn-Schmiedeberg's Arch Pharmacol 1993 (347):506-513

56 Andrews PLR: 5-HT3 receptor antagonists and antiemesis. In: King FC, Jones B and Sanger GJ (eds) 5-HT3 Receptor Antagonists. CRC Press, Boca Raton, USA 1994 pp 255-317

57 Leslie RA and Reynolds DJM: The area postrema and vomiting: how important is serotonin? In: Osborne NN (ed) Current Aspects of the Neurosciences. Macmillan, London 1991 pp 79-101

58 Blackshaw LA and Grundy D: Effects of 5-hydroxytryptamine on discharge of vagal mucosal afferent fibres from the upper gastrointestinal tract of the ferret. J Auton Nerv Syst 1993 (45):41-50

59 Andrews PLR and Davidson HIM: Activation of vagal afferent terminals by 5-hydroxytryptamine is mediated by the 5-HT receptor in the anaesthetized ferret. J Physiol 1990 (422):92P

60 Endo T, Takahashi M, Minami M, Yoshioka M, Saito H, Pavez SH: Effects of anticancer drugs on

enzyme activities and serotonin release from ileal tissue in ferrets. Biogenic Amines 1993 (9):479-489
61 Endo T, Minami M, Monma Y, Saito H, Takeuchi M: Emesis-related biochemical and histopathological changes induced by cisplatin in the ferret. J Toxicol Sci 1990 (15):235-244
62 Fukui H, Yamamoto M, Ando T, Sasaki S, Sato S: Increase in serotonin levels in the dog ileum and blood by cisplatin as measured by microdialysis. Neuropharmacology 1993 (32):959-968
63 Cubeddu LX, Hoffman IS, Fuenmayor NT, Malave JJ: Changes in serotonin metabolism in cancer patients: its relationship to nausea and vomiting induced by chemotherapeutic drugs. Br J Cancer 1992 (66):198-203
64 Barnes NM GeJ, Jones WG, Naylor RJ, Rudd JA: Cisplatin-induced emesis: preliminary results indicative of changes in plasma levels of 5-Hydroxytryptamine. Br J Cancer 1990b (62):862-864
65 Torii Y, Mutoh M, Saito H, Matsuki N: Involvement of free radicals in cisplatin-induced emesis in Suncus murinus. Eur J Pharmacol - Env Toxicol and Pharmacol 1993 (248):131-135
66 Gebauer A, Merger M, Kilbinger H: Modulation by 5-HT3 and 5-HT4 receptors of the release of 5-hydroxytryptamine from the guinea-pig small intestine. Naunyn-Schmiedeberg's Arch Pharmacol 1993 (347):137-140
67 Lee CR, Plosker G, McTavish D: Tropisetron: A review of its pharmacodynamic and pharmacokinetic properties and therapeutic potential as an antiemetic. Drugs 1993 (46):925-943
68 Yarker YE and McTavish D: Granisetron: an update of its therapeutic use in nausea and vomiting induced by antineoplastic therapy. Drugs 1994 (48): 761-793
69 Markham A and Sorkin EM: Ondansetron: An update of its therapeutic use. Drugs 1993 (46/2):268
70 Cubeddu LX: The role of serotonin in chemotherapy-induced emesis in cancer patients. In: Diaz-Rubio E and Martin M (eds) Antiemetic Therapy: Current Status and Future Prospects. Creaciones Elba SA, Madrid 1992 pp 39-56
71 Gunning SJ, Hagan RM, Tyers MB: Cisplatin induces biochemical and histological changes in the small intestine of the ferret. Br J Pharmacol 1987 (90 Suppl):135
72 Allan SG and Smyth JS: Small intestinal mucosal toxicity of cisplatinum. Comparison of toxicity with platinum analogues and dexamethasone. Br J Cancer 1986 (53):355-360
73 Maxwell A, Gaffin SL, Wells MT: Radiotherapy, endotoxins and nausea. Lancet 1986 (1):1148-1149
74 Roos IA, Fairlie DP, Whitehouse MW: A peculiar toxicity manifested by platinum (II) amines in rats: gastric distension after peritoneal administration. Chem Biol Int 1981 (35):111-117
75 Fredrikson M, Hursti T, Furst C-J, Steineck G, Borjeson S, Wikblom M, Peterson C: Nausea in cancer chemotherapy is inversely related to urinary cortisol excretion. Br J Cancer 1992 (65):779-780
76 Rudd JA, Jordan CC, Naylor RJ: Profiles of emetic action of cisplatin in the ferret: a potential model of acute and delayed emesis. Eur J Pharmacol 1994 (262):R1-R2
77 Rudd JA and Naylor RJ: Effects of 5-hydroxytryptamine-3 receptor antagonists on models of acute and delayed emesis induced by cisplatin in the ferret. Neuropharmacol 1994 (33):1607-1608
78 Watson JW, Gonsalves SF, Fossa AJ, McLean S, Seeger T, Andrews PLR: The role of the NK-1 receptor in emetic responses: the anti-emetic effects of CP-99,994 in the ferret and the dog. Br J Pharmacol 1995 (115):84-94
79 Watson JW, Nagahisa A, Lucot J, Andrews PLR: The role of the NK-1 receptor in emetic responses. In: Reynolds DJM, Andrews PLR, Davis CJ (eds) Serotonin and the Scientific Basis of Anti-Emetic Therapy. Oxford Clinical Communications, Oxford 1995 pp 233-239
80 Grelot L, Milano S, Le Stunff H: Does serotonin play a role in the delayed phase of cisplatin-induced emesis? In: Reynolds DJM, Andrews PLR, Davis CJ (eds) Serotonin and the Scientific Basis of Anti-Emetic Therapy. Oxford Clinical Communications, Oxford 1995 pp 181-191
81 Fox RA: Current status: animal models of nausea. In: Bianchi AL, Grelot L, Miller AD, King GL (eds) Mechanisms and Control of Emesis. Colloque INSERM, John Libbey, Eurotext 1992 (223):341-350
82 Blijham GH: Does granisetron remain effective over multiple cycles? Eur J Cancer 1992 (28A Suppl 1):S17-S21
83 Cubeddu LX and Hoffmann IS: Participation of serotonin on early and delayed emesis induced by initial and subsequent cycles of cisplatinum-based chemotherapy: effects of dexamethasone and metoclopramide. J Clin Pharmacol 1993 (33):691-697
84 Andryowski MA: Psychological aspects of nausea and vomiting. In: Bianchi AL, Grelot L, Miller AD, King GL (eds) Mechanisms and Control of Emesis. Colloque INSERM, John Libbey, Eurotext 1992 (223):313-322
85 Morrow GR: The effect of a susceptibility to motion sickness on the side effects of cancer chemotherapy. Cancer 1985 (55):2766-2770
86 Reason JT and Brand JJ: Motion Sickness. Academic Press, London 1975 p 181
87 Palazzo MGA and Strunin L: Anaesthesia and emesis I: Etiology. Can Anaesth Soc J 1984 (31):178-187
88 Palazzo MGA and Strunin L: Anaesthesia and emesis II: Prevention and management. Can Anaesth Soc J 1984 (31):407-415
89 Andrews PLR: Physiology of nausea and vomiting. Br J Anaesth 1992 (69 Suppl 1):2S-19S
90 Begg CB, Cohen JL, Ellerton J: Are the elderly predisposed to toxicity from cancer chemotherapy? Cancer Clin Trials 1980 (3):369-374
91 Morrow GR: Behaviorial factors influencing the development and expression of chemotherapy induced side effects. Br J Cancer 1992 (66):554-561
92 Marr HE, Davey PT, Boyle EA, Blower PB: The anti-emetic activity of granisetron against cytostatic treatment-induced emesis in 10-13 week-old

ferrets. J Cancer Res Clin Oncol 1994 (120):204-207
93 Mirabile CS: Motion sickness susceptibility and behaviour. In: Crampton GH (ed) Motion and Space Sickness. CRC Press, Boca Raton, USA 1990 pp 391-410
94 Miaskiewicz SL, Stricker E, Verbalis JG: Neurohypophyseal secretion in response to cholecystokinin, but not meal-induced gastric distention in human. J Clin Endocrinol Metab 1989 (68):837-843
95 Roila F, Tonato M, Del Favero A: Prognostic factors of chemotherapy-induced emesis. In: Diaz-Rubio E and Martin M (eds) Antiemetic Therapy: Current Status and Future Prospects. Creaciones Elba SA, Madrid 1992
96 Martin M, Diaz-Rubio E: Emesis during past pregnancy: a new prognostic factor in chemotherapy-induced emesis. Ann Oncol 1990 (1):152-153
97 Andrews PLR and Whitehead SA: Pregnancy sickness. News Physiol Sci 1990 (5):5-10
98 Sullivan JR, Leyden MJ, Bell R: Decreased cisplatin-induced nausea and vomiting with chronic alcohol ingestion. N Engl J Med 1983 (309):796
99 Spiess JL, Adelstein DJ, Hines JD: Evaluation of ethanol as an antiemetic in patients receiving cisplatin. Clin Ther 1987 (9):400-404
100 D'Acquisto RW, Tyson LB, Gralla RJ et al: The influence of a chronic high alcohol intake on chemotherapy-induced nausea and vomiting. Proc Am Soc Clin Oncol 1986 (5):257
101 Stern RM, Hu S, LeBlanc R, Koch KL: Chinese hyper-susceptibility to vection-induced motion sickness. Aviat Space Environ Med 1995 (in press)
102 Xu LH, Koch KL, Summy-Long J et al: Hypothalamic and gastric myoelectrical responses during vection-induced nausea in healthy Chinese subjects. Am J Physiol 1993 (265):E578-E584
103 Alfieri AB and Cubeddu LX: Treatment with parachlorophenylalanine antagonises the emetic response and the serotonin-releasing actions of cisplatin in cancer patients. Br J Cancer 1995 (71): 629-632
104 Fink-Jensen A, Judge ME, Hansen JB et al: Inhibition of cisplatin-induced emesis in ferrets by the non-NMDA receptor antagonists NBQX and CNQX. Neurosci Lett 1992 (137):173-177
105 Göthert M, Hamon M, Barann M et al: 5-HT3 receptor antagonism by anpirtoline, a mixed 5-HT1 receptor agonist/5-HT3 receptor antagonist. Br J Pharmacol 1995 (114):269-274
106 Aggarwal SK: A histochemical approach to the mechanism of action of cisplatin and its analogues. J Histochem Cytochem 1993 (41):1053-1073
107 Scott RH, Woods AJ, Lacey MJ, Fernando D, Crawford JH, Andrews PLR: An electrophysiological investigation of the effects of cisplatin and the protective actions of dexamethasone on cultured dorsal root ganglion neurones from neonatal rats. Naunyn-Schmiedeberg's Arch Pharmacol 1995 (352):247-255
108 Roila F: Dexamethasone, granisetron, or both for the prevention of nausea and vomiting during chemotherapy for cancer. New Engl J Med 1995 (332): 1-5
109 Woods AJ and Andrews PLR: Cisplatin acutely reduces 5-HT-induced vagal depolarization in the rat: Protective effect of dexamethasone. Eur J Pharmacol 1995 (278):275-278
110 Aapro MS, Alberts DS, Serokman R: Lack of dexamethasone effect on the antitumour activity of cisplatin. Cancer Treat Rep 1983 (67):1013-1017
111 Maridonneau-Parini I, Errasfa M, Russo-Marie F: Inhibition of O2 generation by dexamethasone is mimicked by lipocortin I in alveolar macrophages. J Clin Invest 1989 (261):395-400

Antiemetic Drugs: Essential Pharmacology

Steven M. Grunberg

Vermont Cancer Center, University of Vermont, Fletcher Allen Health Care, 111 Colchester Avenue - Patrick 534, Burlington, VT 05401-1429, U.S.A.

Development of successful agents and strategies for control of chemotherapy-induced emesis has resulted from a combination of deduction and serendipity. Elucidation of the mechanism of action of various antiemetic agents has led to a better understanding of the physiology upon which the emetic reflex arc is based and this in turn has led to the development of more selective agents with greater efficacy and an improved efficacy/toxicity ratio. However, development of various routes and schedules for antiemetic delivery has also been driven by practical considerations and convenience, and some of the greatest advances have resulted from the lack of selectivity of various antiemetic agents and the resultant identification of additional relevant mechanisms and pathways to serve as targets for antiemetic blockade.

To understand the essential pharmacology of antiemetics, certain fundamental differences between cytotoxic agents and supportive care agents must be appreciated. The field of cytotoxic chemotherapy is still driven to a large extent by the dose-response hypothesis. If a chemotherapeutic agent exhibits antitumour cytotoxic properties, then larger doses of the agent are assumed to exhibit improved antitumour cytotoxic properties. This philosophy has contributed to the increased use of cytokines as supportive care agents for high-dose chemotherapy. This philosophy has also been the driving force behind the development of various permutations of stem cell rescue after marrow ablative therapy (including allogeneic bone marrow transplant, autologous bone marrow transplant, and peripheral blood stem cell infusion).

Antiemetic therapy depends upon a more subtle correlation of emetogenic challenge and antiemetic response. The challenge agents may have differing potencies as emetogens which may require a different level of antiemetic response. In addition, cytotoxic agents are often given as a fixed bolus challenge, resulting in a predictable time course of onset of emetogenic action. Thus different antiemetic agents at greater or lesser doses may be sufficient for the management of emesis induced by various chemotherapeutic agents (with significant pharmacoeconomic implications). Consideration of possible interactions between the mechanism of the antiemetic agent and the mechanism of physiological induction of emesis by the chemotherapeutic agent may also significantly affect the dose and schedule of antiemetic administration.

Binding Affinity and Schedule Dependence

Questions of binding affinity and potency are often raised in discussing the relative efficacy of various antiemetics. In particular the 5-HT_3 antagonists have been compared and characterised in terms of their binding affinity (pK_i) for the 5-HT_3 receptor with the assumption that the frequency and magnitude of significant clinical activity could be deduced. It is certainly true that differences in binding affinity exist among the many members of this family of agents. Even a review of only the most commonly used agents reveals a pK_i for the 5-HT_3 receptor of 8.07 for ondansetron, 8.42 for granisetron, and 8.81 for tropisetron [1]. However, such values cannot be taken in isolation. Although the pK_i values of ondansetron and granisetron do reflect the relative magnitude of the clinically effective doses, the higher pK_i value for tropisetron might be thought to imply an even lower dose for full clinical efficacy. In reality the clinically effective dose of tropisetron is midway between that of ondansetron and that of granisetron. One explanation may lie in further elucidation of the metabolic pathways of these agents. The major (hydroxylated) metabolites of ondansetron have an affinity for the 5-HT_3 receptor that is no more than that of the parent compound [2]. Dolasetron, on the other hand, is rapidly reduced at the ketone group to form a metabolite (MDL 74,156) which has a greater potency as a 5-HT_3 receptor antagonist than the parent compound itself. In fact the (+)-enantiomer of MDL 74,156 (identified as MDL 73,405), which accounts for 90% of the reduced metabolite excreted in urine in human studies, has a pK_i for the 5-HT_3 receptor of 9.12, much higher than any of the commonly used antiserotonergic agents [3]. In spite of this, the required dose of dolasetron for maximum efficacy is greater than that of several other agents [4].

Plasma half-life has also been suggested as a parameter that could be of importance in determining duration of action of various antiemetics. Using the 5-HT_3 antagonists as a model, marked differences in plasma half-life are easily detected. Ondansetron appears to have the shortest half-life of the commonly used 5-HT_3 antagonist antiemetics. Measured values range from 2.5 to 5.5 hours and are directly proportional to age (the reported half-life of ondansetron in subjects 7-12 years old is 2.5 hours [2], for those 18-40 years old 3.2 hours [5], and for those over 75 years old 5.5 hours [6]). However, clearance of ondansetron is decreased in subjects with hepatic insufficiency [2]. By comparison, tropisetron has a plasma half-life of approximately 8 hours [7] while that of granisetron is approximately 11 hours [8]. During the early development of these agents, these differences in half-life led to the development of a multi-dose regimen for ondansetron [9] (3 doses given at 4-hour intervals beginning 30 minutes prior to chemotherapy) for prophylaxis of acute vomiting (vomiting within the first 24 hours after administration of cisplatin) while tropisetron [7] and granisetron [8] were both considered good candidates for single-dose regimens. However, the excellent toxicity profile of the 5-HT_3 antagonists suggested that more flexibility in dose and schedule could be explored in the interest of convenience of administration. An important demonstration of the lack of schedule dependence of a 5-HT_3 antagonist was performed by Marty [10], who randomised 305 patients receiving cisplatin at a dose of at least 50 mg/m^2 to receive a 32 mg dose of intravenous ondansetron either as a single bolus or as an 8 mg loading dose followed by a 1 mg/hr infusion for 24 hours. Antiemetic efficacy was equivalent between the two groups, with 76% of the bolus patients and 72% of the infusion patients achieving complete or major protection from acute emesis. In a similar demonstration, Beck [11] randomised 699 patients receiving either moderate-dose cisplatin (50-70 mg/m^2) or high-dose cisplatin (at least 100 mg/m^2) to receive ondansetron either as a single 8 mg dose, a single 32 mg dose, or in a standard regimen of three 0.15 mg/ kg doses spaced 4 hours apart. The 32 mg single dose was found to be superior to the 8 mg single dose in both the moderate-dose cisplatin and the high-dose cisplatin strata in terms of number of emetic episodes, complete response (no emetic episodes), and failure rate (more than 5 emetic episodes, withdrawn from study, or receiving rescue antiemetics). The 32 mg single dose was also superior to the multi-dose 0.15 mg/kg regimen in terms of number of emetic episodes for the moderate-dose cisplatin stratum and failure rate for both strata. No significant difference in any parameter was found between the 8 mg single dose and the multi-dose 0.15 mg/kg regimen. Since calculation of a 0.15 mg/kg dose for a 70 kg patient results in a dosing regimen of 10.5 mg x 3, it would seem that the 8 mg dose is a reasonable approximation of the first dose of the multi-dose regimen while the 32 mg dose is a reasonable approximation of the cumulative dose of the multi-dose regimen. Thus in spite of the relatively short half-life of ondansetron, the major determinant of response for the full 24 hour period would appear to be the dose of ondansetron administered immediately prior to administration of cisplatin rather than doses designed to provide extended maintenance of ondansetron levels. This would be consistent with the observation by Cubeddu [12] that onset of cisplatin-induced emesis and maximum excretion of urinary 5-HIAA both appear within the first 6 hours after administration of cisplatin, suggesting again that intervention before and during the emetogenic challenge is the primary determinant of efficacy for the entire acute eme-

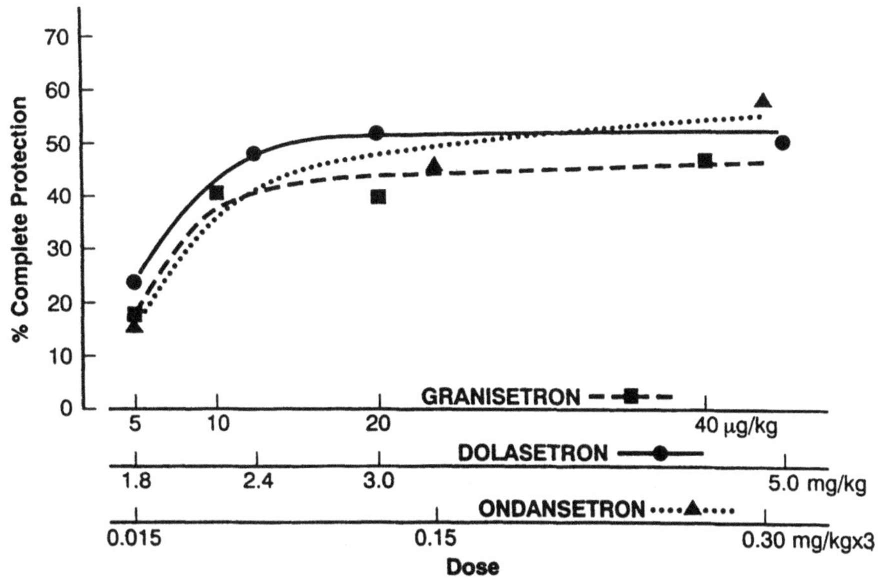

Fig. 1. Similar relationship between complete protection from emesis induced by high-dose cisplatin and dose for the 5-HT_3 antagonists ondansetron, granisetron and dolasetron. Adapted from Kris [4], Grunberg [13], and Navari [14]

sis period.

More striking than the differences between the various 5-HT_3 antiemetics has been their clinical similarity in both efficacy and toxicity. All of these agents have been characterised by an excellent toxicity profile, with mild headache being the most common toxicity and alterations in bowel function, hepatic function, or alertness appearing at higher doses [4,13,14]. The correlation between dose and antiemetic efficacy has also followed a similar pattern. Although the minimum fully effective dose against emesis from high-dose cisplatin has differed (approximately 0.01 mg/kg for granisetron, 2 mg/kg for dolasetron, and 0.05 mg/kg x 3 for ondansetron), the pattern of a rapid slope of dose-response until the effective dose is reached followed by a relative plateau in efficacy as dose is increased further has been remarkably reproducible (Fig. 1). This pattern might suggest a threshold value at which full saturation of the relevant receptor is achieved (although 100% efficacy is still not achieved).

Various schedules of administration have also been studied with other antiemetic families. Extended infusion of antidopaminergic antiemetics has been viewed as both a method to increase overall efficacy and a method to decrease toxicity. Extended infusion schedules for both metoclopramide and prochlorperazine have therefore been studied. Taylor [15] has administered metoclopramide in doses up to 10 mg/kg (5 mg/kg loading dose followed by a 0.66 mg/kg infusion x 8 hours) while Carr [16] administered prochlorperazine as a 30 mg loading dose followed by infusion at doses up to 20 mg/hr x 24 hours accompanied by bolus diphenhydramine. Although all of these various infusion regimens were found to be tolerable, none suggested efficacy superior to that of a bolus regimen of the same agent.

Routes of Administration

Although the intravenous route is the most predictable in terms of drug delivery and bioavailabilty, this route is only practical in the inpatient setting. Since chemotherapy is increasingly being given in the outpatient setting and extended administration of antiemetics to respond to the possibility of recurrent or continuing emesis is desirable, a number of other routes have been explored. The oral route has been by far the most popular. Most of the traditional antiemetic families can be successfully administered by the oral route. Such agents would include the phenothiazines, butyrophenones, substituted benzamides, and cannabinoids, as well as ancillary agents such as the antihistamines and benzodiazepines. Both licensed (ondansetron [17], granisetron [18]) and investigational (RS 42358-197 [19] and pancopride [20]) 5-HT_3 antagonists have also been shown to be effective when administered orally.

The oral route has significant intrinsic limitations,

including questions of absorption and effect of first-pass hepatic clearance on bioavailability. Bateman [21] emphasized the wide interpatient variation of bioavailability of standard doses (10 mg or 20 mg) of oral metoclopramide. Although the mean bioavailability in 7 patients was 61%, individual bioavailability ranged from 32% to 97%, making prospective determination of appropriate doses difficult. Administration of high-dose metoclopramide (2.5 mg/kg/dose) increased the bioavailability to 87% but was still associated with a significant variability in individual values (65% to 118%) [22]. Although oral ondansetron is almost completely absorbed, bioavailability is only about 60%, suggesting 40% first-pass metabolism in the liver [23]. The bioavailability of oral granisetron is also about 60% [24]. Prochlorperazine has been noted to have a bioavailability of less than 16% when administered orally [25] while the bioavailability of oral tetrahydrocannabinol is only 10% to 20% [26]. In the case of metoclopramide the additional question of changes in toxicity profile has been raised [27], with the suggestion that an increased incidence of dystonic reactions may be seen with oral metoclopramide.

The oral route also has a number of disadvantages specific to the setting of prevention of chemotherapy-induced emesis. In a situation where prevention of emesis is much more effective than rescue treatment of acute emesis and development of anticipatory emesis is highly dependent on previous experience [28], it is extremely important that reliable and effective doses of antiemetics be delivered during even the first course of chemotherapy, without adjustment for interpatient variability. In cases where efficacy of the initial antiemetic dose is insufficient, the act of vomiting itself may make delivery and retention of further oral antiemetic doses difficult. In addition, continuous nausea during chemotherapy or anticipatory nausea after a poor experience with previous chemotherapy may limit patient compliance with an oral regimen. Several alternative routes have therefore been proposed to avoid hepatic metabolism while maintaining ease of administration and high rates of absorption.

To continue to use the alimentary tract, both rectal and buccal routes have been investigated. Some antiemetics, such as prochlorperazine, have long been available in the form of rectal suppositories. Mattes [29] has also investigated the potential role of this route in administration of cannabinoids, particularly for patients with demonstrated low plasma levels of cannabinoid after oral administration. Plasma pharmacokinetics in 3 patients receiving tetrahydrocannabinol in doses equivalent to those used for oral administration were measured and revealed a 30-fold increase in cannabinoid plasma exposure (area under the curve) after rectal administration. Cannabinoids are also well absorbed through the bronchial mucosa, with bioavailability 5 to 10-fold greater than the oral route [30]. In a single-arm study, Vinciguerra [31] administered tetrahydrocannabinol by inhalation to 56 patients who were refractory to conventional antiemetics. A 78% response rate was observed (self-rating by patients of the antiemetic efficacy of tetrahydrocannabinol as very effective or moderately effective). The buccal route has been studied as an alternative for administration of prochlorperazine in the post-operative setting. Patterson [32] randomised 52 female patients undergoing gynaecological surgery or breast biopsy to receive no antiemetic or 6 mg prochlorperazine as buccal tablets 1 hr before surgery and observed a reduction in the incidence of nausea from 58% to 15%.

Transdermal administration would appear to be another route that would be non-invasive and could maintain significant exposure to antiemetics. Transdermal scopolamine, for example, has been quite successful in the treatment of motion sickness [33] and also has been suggested to have efficacy as an adjuvant agent for chemotherapy-induced emesis [34]. Calpena [35] therefore studied a series of clinically used antiemetics including phenothiazines, butyrophenones, and substituted benzamides in a rat skin model to determine parameters of transdermal penetrance in comparison to scopolamine. Melting point and apparent partition coefficient of the antiemetic were found to be significantly correlated with transdermal permeability rate. However, only one of the test agents studied (bromopride) was predicted to achieve a steady-state concentration within the therapeutic range, and the problem of delayed lag time until steady state is reached by this route was also noted.

Novel Neurotransmitter Receptors

Over the last several decades, advances in antiemetic therapy have been driven by the need to counteract the effects of increasingly emetogenic chemotherapy. However, quantum increases in antiemetic efficacy have been achieved when new relevant neurotransmitter receptors have been identified and appropriate antagonists have been synthesized. Identification of 5-HT_3 receptor antagonism as a secondary effect of high-dose metoclopramide was instrumental in the development of clinical interest in this new mechanism. Ironically, identification of a new receptor is inevitably followed by emphasis on increasing specificity of receptor blockade by new antiemetic agents. Even the present generation of supposedly specific 5-HT_3 antagonists may show some affinity for other receptors and processes. Ondansetron, for example, also binds the 5-HT_{1B}, 5-HT_{1C}, α1-adrenergic, and μ-opiate receptors, while tropisetron affects 5-HT uptake [1]. It should be remembered that no single agent identified to date produces reliable complete protection in 100% of patients receiving highly emetogenic chemotherapy. Thus either the ultimate mechanism of emetogenesis has not yet been identified or emesis is the result of multiple potential neuronal pathways that will require combinations of effective blocking agents with different neurophysiological targets.

Several additional neurotransmitter receptors have now been suggested as having a possible role in chemotherapy-induced emesis. Kobrinsky [36], for example, demonstrated that administration of naloxone even in the absence of specific opiate challenge could increase the emetogenicity of chemotherapy, suggesting an antiemetic role for endogenous opiate agonists and receptors. However, the contradictory effects of morphine itself, which can function either as an emetic agonist or antagonist under appropriate conditions, made development of effective agents more difficult. Work with more specific agents, such as the potent μ-receptor agonist fentanyl, has provided a more consistent explanation. Fentanyl [37] is not emetogenic itself but can antagonise morphine-induced emesis. Emetic protection induced by fentanyl can itself be reversed by naloxone. Localization of the μ receptor in the nucleus tractus solitarius and area postrema adds further support to the role of this receptor in emetic pathways. Thus it is currently suggested that the δ or κ opiate receptors may serve as mediators of emetogenesis while the μ receptor serves as a mediator of antiemesis, opening the way to development of clinically effective agents from this family. Two other substances of potential interest are plasma peptide YY (PYY) and Substance P. Perry [38] has suggested that plasma levels of PYY are more strongly correlated with cisplatin-induced emesis and antiemetic protection than are plasma levels of 5-HT, indicating a possible independent or complementary role in induction of emesis. Substance P is generally considered to be a mediator of nociception [39]. Although Substance P can act as a modulator of serotonergic activity, the mechanism of emetic/antiemetic activity of this compound is less certain. Resinferatoxin, a highly potent capsaicin analogue which causes transient depletion of Substance P and does not activate the Bezold-Jarisch reflex, has been shown to have antiemetic properties against both chemical- and radiation-induced emesis in the ferret [40]. In addition, synthetic antagonists of the NK-1 receptor, the target of Substance P, have also been suggested to have antiemetic activity [41]. Thus the Substance P pathway may provide new antiemetic agents that can complement or be used independently of currently available agents.

Modulation of Receptors

Modulation of the sensitivity or concentration of relevant neurotransmitter receptors could also alter the balance of emetogenicity, leading to new strategies for antiemetic control and for identification of particularly sensitive (or resistant) subjects. Blum [42] and Cloninger [43] both noted a higher prevalence of the A1 allele of the dopamine D_2 receptor gene in alcoholics as compared to non-alcoholic controls. Analysis of brain tissue revealed a lower concentration (but not affinity) of dopamine D_2 receptors in subjects carrying the A1 as compared to the A2 allele [44]. Since dopaminergic reward pathways may be involved in the establishment of addictive behaviour [45], the ability of alcohol-induced increases in brain dopamine to more easily saturate pathways in A1 allele-carrying subjects might explain an increased tendency toward alcoholism. By the same token, greater saturation of the less numerous dopamine D_2 receptors encoded by the A1 allele either by emetogenic mediators or by antiemetic agents or their metabolites could result in a differing susceptibility to chemotherapy-induced emesis in these individuals. The well-described association between a history of significant alcohol intake and decreased risk of chemotherapy-induced emesis [46-48] might therefore have a physiological basis in differing expression of the pharmacological target.

When 5-HT_3 antagonists are used at a fixed dose during administration of a 5-day course of cisplatin, a gradual decrease in antiemetic efficacy is noted. Loss of efficacy could result from a combination of repeated induction of acute vomiting, appearance of delayed vomiting, and development of anticipatory vomiting during the treatment period. However, induced modulation of relevant neurotransmitter receptors would provide an equally plausible explanation. Upregulation (expression of an increased number or density of receptors (B_{max}) without a change in receptor affinity (K_d)) has already been described for numerous members of the 5-HT receptor family. In brain tissue an increase in 5-HT_{1A} [49], 5-HT_{1B} [50], and 5-HT_{1C} [51] receptors has been noted with ethanol exposure or chemical axotomy. An increase in 5-HT_2 [52] receptors on platelet membranes has been associated with transformed migraine headaches. The suggestion that loss of antiemetic control during multi-day cisplatin-based chemotherapy might result from upregulation of 5-HT_3 receptors due to either chemotherapy exposure or antiemetic exposure provides both an explanation and a testable hypothesis. If this hypothesis is correct, daily escalation of 5-HT_3 receptor antagonist dose might prevent the development of antiemetic resistance by matching a pharmacological strategy to a physiological response.

Modulation of neurotransmitter pathways relevant to the antiemetic response may also take place through activation of other similarly relevant pathways. The dual activity of high-dose metoclopramide in both antidopaminergic and antiserotonergic pathways is perhaps the best demonstration of clinically relevant interactions. However, the finding by Brann [53] using target size analysis that the serotonin-S_2 and dopamine-D_2 receptors in rat brain membranes are of similar size may suggest one mechanism for interaction between serotonergic and dopaminergic pathways. In addition, several examples of serotonergic regulation of dopamine-related neural activity have been described, including regulation of carbaryl-induced tremor [54], regulation of nigrostriatal neurons [55], and modulation of 3,4-methylenedioxymethamphetamine neurotoxicity [56]. Zhou [57] observed sprouting and dense growth of serotonergic fibres in the rat substantia nigra and striatum after dopaminergic denervation, while Hagan [58] found that ondansetron could inhibit both the hyperactivity and the increased dopamine metabolism induced by injection of DiMe-C7 into the ventral tegmental area of the rat brain. Another particularly intriguing interaction has been suggested through study of the chicken ovalbumin upstream promoter transcription factor, a member of the steroid receptor superfamily. Power [59] has described activation of this gene by physiological concentrations of dopamine and by the dopamine receptor agonist ergocryptine. Thus the clinical interaction between corticosteroids and antidopaminergic agents could have a basis in activation of as yet unidentified common pathways. Even newly identified emetogenic neurotransmitters may prove to act in part through modulation of previously recognised pathways. Rawdon [60] has described cross-reactivity of a Substance P antiserum with serotonin, raising the possibility of physiological cross-reaction. In the spinal cord, denervation supersensitivity to 5-HT may depend on a concurrent absence of Substance P [61]. Conversely, various 5-HT receptors may affect transmission of nociceptive information [62]. Activation of peripheral 5-HT_3 receptors, for example, may increase transmission of such information [63] while activation of spinal cord 5-HT_3 receptors will reduce transmission [64].

The essential pharmacology of antiemetic management is not merely a matter of achievement of appropriate plasma peak level or exposure duration since these parameters have shown little correlation with antiemetic efficacy [65]. The complex nature of the emetogenic pathways provides an ever-increasing range of independent and interdependent neurotransmitter receptor targets. Exploration of new routes of administration and new receptor targets will increase the therapeutic armamentarium, while modulation of these receptors may prove to be as important as blockade of the receptors themselves. Greater understanding of these different pathways and their physiological interactions will therefore allow more sophisticated administration of currently available agents and of newly developed agents to achieve greater overall efficacy with better patient acceptance and improved quality of life.

REFERENCES

1 Van Wijngaarden I, Tulp MTM, Soudijn W: The concept of selectivity in 5-HT receptor research. Eur J Pharmacol 1990 (188):301-312

2 Pritchard JF: Ondansetron metabolism and pharmacokinetics. Semin Oncol 1992 (19 Suppl 10):9-15

3 Bigaud M, Elands J, Kastner PR, Bohnke RA, Emmert LW, Galvan M: Pharmacology of the human metabolites of dolasetron, an antiemetic 5-HT3 receptor antagonist. Drug Dev Res 1995 (34):289-296

4 Kris MG, Grunberg SM, Gralla RJ, Baltzer L, Zaretsky SA, Lifsey D, Tyson LB, Schmidt L, Hahne WF: Dose-ranging evaluation of the serotonin antagonist dolasetron mesylate in patients receiving high-dose cisplatin. J Clin Oncol 1994 (12):1045-1049

5 Colthup PV, Felgate CC, Plamer JL, Scully NL: Determination of ondansetron in plasma and its pharmacokinetics in the young and elderly. J Pharm Sci 1991 (80):868-871

6 Pritchard JF, Bryson JC, Kernodle AE, Benedetti TL, Powell JR: Age and gender effects on ondansetron pharmacokinetics: evaluation of healthy aged volunteers. Clin Pharmacol Ther 1992 (51):51-55

7 Lee CR, Plosker GL, McTavish D: Tropisetron - a review of its pharmacodynamic and pharmacokinetic properties, and therapeutic potential as an antiemetic. Drugs 1993 (46):925-943

8 Addelman M, Erlichman C, Fine S, Warr D, Murray C: Phase I/II trial of granisetron: a novel 5-hydroxytryptamine antagonist for the prevention of chemotherapy-induced nausea and vomiting. J Clin Oncol 1990 (8):337-341

9 Grunberg SM, Stevenson LL, Russell CA, McDermed JE: Dose ranging phase I study of the serotonin antagonist GR38032F for prevention of cisplatin-induced nausea and vomiting. J Clin Oncol 1989 (7):1137-1141

10 Marty M, d'Allens H and Groupe Multicentrique Français: Etude randomisée en double-insu comparant l'efficacité de l'ondansetron selon deux modes d'administration: injection unique et perfusion continue. Cahiers Cancer 1990 (2):541-546

11 Beck TM, Hesketh PJ, Madajewicz S et al: Stratified, randomized, double-blind comparison of intravenous ondansetron administered as a multiple-dose regimen versus two single-dose regimens in the prevention of cisplatin-induced nausea and vomiting. J Clin Oncol 1991 (10):1969-1975

12 Cubeddu LX, Hoffman IS, Fuenmayor NT, Finn AL: Efficacy of ondansetron (GR38032F) and the role of serotonin in cisplatin-induced nausea and vomiting. N Engl J Med 1990 (322):810-816

13 Grunberg SM, Lane M, Lester EP, Sridhar KS, Mortimer J, Murphy W, Sanderson PE: Randomized double-blind comparison of three dose levels of intravenous ondansetron in the prevention of cisplatin-induced emesis. Cancer Chemother Pharmacol 1993 (32):268-272

14 Navari RM, Kaplan HG, Gralla RJ, Grunberg SM, Palmer R, Fitts D: Efficacy and safety of granisetron, a selective 5-hydroxytryptamine-3 receptor antagonist, in the prevention of nausea and vomiting induced by high-dose cisplatin. J Clin Oncol 1994 (12):2204-2210

15 Taylor WB, Simpson JM, Bateman DN: High-dose metoclopramide by infusion: a double-blind study of plasma concentration-effect relationships in patients receiving cancer chemotherapy. Eur J Clin Pharmacol 1987 (33):161-165

16 Carr BI, Morgan R, Doroshow JH, Raschko J, Leong L, Margolin K, Somlo A, Akman S: Phase I clinical study of 24 hr continuous infusion prochlorperazine (compazine). Proc Am Soc Clin Oncol 1990 (9):324

17 Fraschini G, Ciociola A, Esparza L, Templeton D, Holmes FA, Walters RS, Hortobagyi GN: Evaluation of three oral dosages of ondansetron in the prevention of nausea and emesis associated with cyclophosphamide-doxorubicin chemotherapy. J Clin Oncol 1991 (9):1268-1274

18 Hacking A: Oral granisetron - simple and effective: a preliminary report. Eur J Cancer 1992 (28A Suppl 1): S28-S32

19 Eglen RM, Lee CH, Smith WL, Johnson LG, Whiting RL, Hedge SS: RS 42358-197, a novel and potent 5-HT3 receptor antagonist, in vitro and in vivo. J Pharmacol Exp Ther 1993 (266):535-543

20 Fernández AG, Puig J, Beleta J, Doménech T, Bou J, Berga P, Gristwood RW, Roberts DJ: Pancopride, a potent and long-acting 5-HT3 receptor antagonist, is orally effective against anticancer drug-evoked emesis. Eur J Pharmacol 1992 (222):257-264

21 Bateman DN, Kahn C, Davies DS: The pharmacokinetics of metoclopramide in man with observations in the dog. Br J Clin Pharmacol 1980 (9):371-377

22 Taylor WB and Bateman DN: Oral bioavailability of high-dose metoclopramide. Eur J Clin Pharmacol 1986 (31):41-44

23 Saynor DA and Dixon CM: The metabolism of ondansetron. Eur J Cancer Clin Oncol 1989 (25 Suppl 1): S75-S77

24 Cupissol D, Bressolle F, Adenis L, Carmichael J, Bessell E, Allen A, Wargenau M, Romain D: Evaluation of the bioequivalence of tablet and capsule formulations of granisetron in patients undergoing cytotoxic chemotherapy for malignant disease. J Pharm Sci 1993 (82):1281-1284

25 Taylor WB and Bateman DN: Preliminary studies of the pharmacokinetics and pharmacodynamics of prochlorperazine in healthy volunteers. Br J Clin Pharmacol 1987 (23):137-142

26 Wall ME, Sadler BM, Brine D, Taylor H, Parez-Reyes M: Metabolism, disposition, and kinetics of delta-9-

tetrahydrocannabinol in men and women. Clin Pharmacol Ther 1983 (34):352-363
27 Tyson LB, Gralla RJ, Kris MG, Young CS, Clark RA: Dose-ranging antiemetic trial of high-dose oral metoclopramide. Am J Clin Oncol 1989 (12):239-243
28 Morrow GR, Lindke JL, Black PM: Predicting development of anticipatory nausea in cancer patients: prospective examination of eight clinical characteristics. J Pain Symptom Manage 1991 (6):215-223
29 Mattes RD, Shaw LM, Edling-Owens J, Engelman K, Elsohly MA: Bypassing the first-pass effect for the therapeutic use of cannabinoids. Pharmacol Biochem Behav 1993 (44):745-747
30 Nahas GG: Current status of marijuana research. JAMA 1979 (242):2775-2778
31 Vinciguerra V, Moore T, Brennan E: Inhalation marijuana as an antiemetic for cancer chemotherapy. NY State J Med 1988 (88):525-527
32 Patterson WK and Keane PW: Use of the buccal route for the administration of an antiemetic. Anesth Analg 1992 (74):937-938
33 Clissold SP and Heel RC: Transdermal hyoscine (scopolamine) - a preliminary review of its pharmacodynamic properties and therapeutic efficacy. Drugs 1985 (29):189-207
34 Meyer BR, O'Mara V, Reidenberg MM: A controlled clinical trial of the addition of transdermal scopolamine to a standard metoclopramide and dexamethasone antiemetic regimen. J Clin Oncol 1987 (5): 1994-1997
35 Calpena AC, Blanes C, Moreno J, Obach R, Domenech J: A comparative *in vitro* study of transdermal absorption of antiemetics. J Pharm Sci 1994 (83):29-33
36 Kobrinsky NL, Pruden PB, Cheang MS, Levitt M, Bishop AJ, Tenenbein M: Increased nausea and vomiting induced by naloxone in patients receiving cancer chemotherapy. Am J Pediatr Hematol Oncol 1988 (10):206-208
37 Barnes NM, Bunce KT, Naylor RJ, Rudd JA: The actions of fentanyl to inhibit drug-induced emesis. Neuropharmacology 1991 (30):1073-1083
38 Perry MR, Rhee J, Smith WL: Plasma levels of peptide YY correlate with cisplatin-induced emesis in dogs. J Pharm Pharmacol 1994 (46):553-557
39 Yaksh TL, Jessell TM, Gamse R, Mudge AW, Leeman SE: Intrathecal morphine inhibits substance P release from mammalian spinal cord *in vivo.* Nature 1980 (286):155-157
40 Andrews PLR and Bhandari P: Resinferatoxin, an ultrapotent capsaicin analogue, has antiemetic properties in the ferret. Neuropharmacology 1993 (32):799-806
41 Bountra C, Bunce K, Dale T, Gardner C, Jordan C, Twissell D, Ward P: Antiemetic profile of a nonpeptide neurokinin NK_1 receptor antagonist, CP-99,994, in ferrets. Eur J Pharmacol 1993 (249):R3-4
42 Blum K, Noble EP, Sheridan PJ et al: Allelic association of human dopamine D_2 receptor gene in alcoholism. JAMA 1990 (263):2055-2060
43 Cloninger CR: D2 dopamine receptor gene is associated but not linked with alcoholism. JAMA 1991 (266):1833-1834
44 Noble EP, Blum K, Ritchie T, Montgomery A, Sheridan PJ: Allelic association of the D_2 dopamine receptor gene with receptor binding characteristics in alcoholism. Arch Gen Psychiatry 1991 (48):648-654
45 Wise RA and Rompre PP: Brain dopamine and reward. Ann Rev Psychol 1989 (40):191-225
46 Sullivan JR, Leyden MJ, Bell R: Decreased cisplatin induced nausea and vomiting with alcohol ingestion. N Engl J Med 1983 (309):796
47 D'Acquisto RW, Tyson LB, Gralla RJ, Clark RA, Kris MG, Von Witte DM, Cacavio A: The influence of a chronic high alcohol intake on chemotherapy-induced nausea and vomiting. Proc Am Soc Clin Oncol 1985 (5):257
48 Hesketh PJ, Murphy WK, Lester EP et al: GR38032F (GR-C507/75): a novel compound effective in the prevention of acute cisplatin-induced emesis. J Clin Oncol 1989 (7):700-705
49 Wong DT, Reid LR, Li TK, Lumeng L: Greater abundance of serotonin$_{1A}$ receptor in some brain areas of alcohol-preferring rats compared to non-preferring rats. Pharmacol Biochem Behav 1993 (46):173-177
50 Manrique C, Segu L, Héry F, Héry M, Faudon M, Franois-Bellan AM: Increase of central 5-HT$_{1B}$ binding sites following 5,7-dihydroxytryptamine axotomy in the adult rat. Brain Res 1993 (623):345-348
51 Pandey SC, Dubey MP, Piano MR, Schwertz DW, Davis JM, Pandey GN: Modulation of 5-HT$_{1C}$ receptors and phosphoinositide system by ethanol consumption in rat brain and choroid plexus. Eur J Pharmacol 1993 (247):81-88
52 Srikiatkhachorn A, Govitrapong P, Limthavon C: Upregulation of 5-HT2 serotonin receptor: a possible mechanism of transformed migraine. Headache 1994 (34):8-11
53 Brann, MR: Serotonin-S2 and dopamine-D2 receptors are the same size in membranes. Biochem Biophys Res Commun 1985 (133):1181-1186
54 Ray SK and Poddar MK: Interaction of central serotonin and dopamine in the regulation of carbaryl-induced tremor. Eur J Pharmacol 1990 (181):159-166
55 Kelland MD, Freeman AS, Chiodo LA: Serotonergic afferent regulation of the basic physiology and pharmacological responsiveness of nigrostriatal dopamine neurons. J Pharmacol Exp Ther 1990 (253):803-811
56 Schmidt CJ, Taylor VL, Abbate GM, Nieduzak TR: 5-HT2 antagonists stereoselectively prevent the neurotoxicity of 3,4-methylenedioxymethamphetamine by blocking the acute stimulation of dopamine synthesis: reversal by L-dopa. J Pharmacol Exp Ther 1991 (256):230-235
57 Zhou FC, Bledsoe S, Murphy J: Serotonergic sprouting is induced by dopamine-lesion in substantia nigra of adult rat brain. Brain Res 1991 (556):108-116
58 Hagan RM, Butler A, Hill JM, Jordan CC, Ireland SJ, Tyers MB: Effect of the 5-HT3 receptor antagonist, GR38032F, on responses to injection of a neurokinin agonist into the ventral tegmental area of the rat brain. Eur J Pharmacol 1987 (138):303-305
59 Power RF, Lydon JP, Conneely OM, O'Malley BW: Dopamine activation of an orphan of the steroid receptor superfamily. Science 1991 (252):1546-1548

60 Rawdon BB and Andrew A: Distribution of serotonin-immunoreactive gut endocrine cells in mice: differential effects on the sensitivity to 5-MeODMT, 8-OH-DPAT and 5-HTP as measured by two nociceptive tests. Brain Res 1988 (440):42-52

62 Eide PK and Hole K: The role of 5-hydroxytryptamine (5-HT) receptor subtypes and plasticity in the 5-HT systems in the regulation of nociceptive sensitivity. Cephalalgia 1993 (13):75-85

63 Eschalier A, Kayser V, Guilbaud G: Influence of a specific 5-HT3 antagonist on carrageenan-induced hyperalgesia in rats. Pain 1989 (36):249-255

64 Alhaider AA, Lei SZ, Wilcox GL: Spinal 5-HT3 receptor-mediated antinociception: possible release of GABA. J Neurosci 1991 (11):1881-1888

65 Campbell M and Bateman DN: Pharmacokinetic optimisation of antiemetic therapy. Clin Pharmacokinet 1992 (23):147-160

Methodology of Antiemetic Trials

Enzo Ballatori [1], Fausto Roila [2] and Albano Del Favero [3]

1 Medical Statistics Unit, Department of Internal Medicine and Public Health, University of L'Aquila
2 Medical Oncology Division, Policlinico Monteluce, Via Brunamonti, 06122 Perugia
3 Institute of Internal Medicine and Oncological Sciences, Policlinico Monteluce, Via Brunamonti, 06122 Perugia, Italy

The aim of this chapter is to outline the specific issues encountered in designing and analysing data from clinical trials on the antiemetic efficacy and tolerability of therapies in cancer patients receiving chemotherapy. This is necessary not only to obtain optimal control of systematic errors, but also to describe their influence on the statistical analysis of the responses.

Nausea and vomiting induced by antineoplastic agents are extremely variable phenomena, depending not only on observable characteristics, whether therapy or patient related, but also on a subjective feeling excited by the impact of the care system on the patient's individual situation. Therefore, in the presence of such high variability, large comparative trials should be carried out to obtain representative and reliable results allowing identification of the most efficacious antiemetic regimens.

In this field, some of the main problems arising in all clinical trials have their own specificity, and our attention will be focussed on these aspects: study design, follow-up and the importance of the prognostic factors. In addition, three topics must clearly be highlighted: the definition of the response variables, the phenomenon of delayed emesis and the assessment of variability of the results obtained with the same antiemetic regimen from one cycle of chemotherapy to the following (i.e., persistence).

Response Variables

Generally, nausea and vomiting, which refer to two different (from a physiopathological point of view) although not uncorrelated phenomena, are evaluated separately.

Chemotherapy-induced nausea and vomiting are currently distinguished in acute and delayed emesis. Acute emesis (nausea or vomiting) is that which the patient experiences in the 24-hour interval after chemotherapy administration, whereas delayed emesis refers to subsequent days. This distinction is based on the fact that in early studies, when really efficacious antiemetic therapies were not available, acute emesis was more often present and more severe than delayed emesis. The distinction also exists because the physiopathological mechanisms are probably different, although those producing delayed emesis (which is absent in animal models) are not yet clearly understood.

Two main aspects of both nausea and vomiting should be evaluated separately: 1) protection from emesis and 2) severity (or intensity) of emesis in patients who did experience emesis. Moreover, in these latter patients, the time to onset of emesis from the instant of chemotherapy administration can also give useful information about the dynamics of emesis. More difficult to evaluate is the duration of emesis, i.e., the time interval in which the patient suffers from emesis.

Vomiting

Vomiting episodes and retches are generally not considered as different since both refer to the same phenomenon.

Protection from acute vomiting is traditionally distinguished as [1]:

- complete protection from vomiting: no vomiting episode (or retch);
- major protection: one or two emetic episodes;
- minor protection: from 3 to 5 emetic episodes.

When a patient has more than 5 emetic episodes, this is considered as a Failure.

Because of the availability of efficacious antiemetic treatments, mainly with moderately emetogenic chemotherapies, we believe only two responses can be considered:

- complete protection from vomiting, as the only positive response (success) of antiemetic prophylaxis;
- failure, in the case of 3 or more emetic episodes. In fact, in many clinical trials, a rescue treatment can be assigned after the third emetic episode.

The severity of emesis can be measured by counting the emetic episodes (or retches), which must be separated by at least one-minute intervals to make sure that one prolonged emetic episode is not interpreted as a number of distinct episodes.

Obviously, the mean number of emetic episodes must be evaluated only in patients who experienced emesis; otherwise, its level could be strongly conditioned by complete protection from vomiting which instead is assumed to be a measurement of a different dimension of efficacy.

Analogously, the time to onset of vomiting should be evaluated only in patients who vomited, also because, in this case, its median should always be calculated and no censored value is to be considered.

In conclusion, at least two parameters should be used to explore the different dimensions of acute vomiting with the aim of evaluating the efficacy of an antiemetic treatment: 1) the percentage of complete protection from vomiting and 2) the mean number of emetic episodes in patients who experienced emesis. Two additional indices could be used to obtain interesting information: 1) the percentage of failure (generally correlated with the mean number of emetic episodes) and 2) the mean time to onset of emesis, to improve our knowledge of the dynamic aspects of vomiting.

To evaluate delayed emesis on a daily basis, the same indices could be used, whereas for a global evaluation (for instance, days 2-5) only percentages of complete protection (or failure) should be used to assess the efficacy of the antiemetic treatment. This is because of the difficulty in interpreting the mean number of emetic episodes, which could refer to many patients who had a small number of emetic episodes in a few days as well as to a few patients who vomited during many days.

Nausea

Complete protection from nausea is the widest used criterion to evaluate the efficacy of antiemetic regimens against this phenomenon. However, the severity of nausea can also be measured. There are several scales available for this:

- Descriptive ordinal Scales (DS), generally used with a 4-level score (0 = no nausea; 1 = mild nausea which does not interfere with normal daily life; 2 = moderate nausea which interferes with normal daily life; 3 = severe nausea, patient bedridden because of nausea);
- Visual Analogue Scales (VAS), i.e., a 100 mm long horizontal line with the extremes marked as '"no nausea" and "worst nausea I have ever felt", with no intermediate divisions or descriptive terms. A score from 0-100 is obtained by measuring the distance from the extreme indicated as "no nausea" to the mark placed by patient along the line;
- Analogue Continuous Chromatic Scales (ACCS), consisting of a 100 mm long and 25 mm wide coloured horizontal bar (from pale pink to red), containing no marking except for the anchor points at each end: "no nausea" (left), "worst nausea" (right).

A substantial equivalence of these three scales has been shown in a study comparing their reliability and responsiveness [2].

More interestingly, whichever scale is used, it is possible to define more dimensions of intensities of nausea. The most common is the maximal intensity of nausea, defined as the highest value of the score obtained with a descriptive or analogue scale at any evaluation performed over the observation time. The entity (the sum of all intensities recorded at each evaluation time) and quantity (the sum of the products of the intensity by the duration, both recorded at each evaluation) could also be

used to assess the severity of nausea.
Although quantity was found to be the most sensitive dimension [2], there proved to be good agreement among these modalities of evaluation. This prompted us to suggest, according to the principle of maximal simplicity, the use of the maximal intensity of nausea, evaluated by a 4-level DS [1].

Mixed Responses

Nausea and vomiting are not independent phenomena. Nevertheless, there are some patients who have nausea without emetic episodes and others who suffer from vomiting but not from nausea. In this case, as is well known in epidemiological research, the analysis of the two phenomena carried out independently could be misleading because of the correlation effects. While the study of such dependence effect will be discussed in the efficacy analysis section of this chapter, here it has to be remembered that to avoid these difficulties in interpreting the results from a clinical trial, some authors suggest evaluating a unique response, mixing the two outcomes, and considering as "success" the absence of both nausea and vomiting (or complete protection from vomiting and nausea at most mild) [3,4].
We disagree with these suggestions mainly because of the dependence of nausea and vomiting on different physiopathological mechanisms. First of all, if we consider a unique response we would be unable to distinguish different efficacy of the antiemetic treatment on nausea or vomiting. Moreover, there are differences in their effects on individual patients: non-prolonged mild or moderate nausea could be preferred by some patients to one or a few emetic episodes, while for others prolonged nausea would be worse than a few emetic episodes. Finally, if a mixed response is considered the risk exists that people who are in quite different conditions will be classified under the same label. For example, a patient could be classified as a "failure" if he had moderate short-term nausea but was protected against vomiting, and so could a patient who had no nausea but suffered many emetic episodes.
In conclusion, we believe that nausea and vomiting should be evaluated separately, without forgetting to analyse their relationship.

Prognostic Factors

Without considering the random errors, the response, i.e., what is assessed in each subject at the end of the experiment, depends not only on the antiemetic therapy administered but on many other, often interrelated variables. These are called prognostic factors and they can be classified as either related to chemotherapy or to patient population. They should be carefully taken into account in planning a clinical trial as well as in analysing its results. In fact, the importance of one or a few prognostic factors can sometimes cause a modification in the study design (e.g., stratifying the patients before randomisation). Moreover, when analysing data, different efficacy between treatments could be found stronger or weaker in patient subsets defined by a particular combination of levels of prognostic factors, and this could have great importance from a clinical point of view.
As concerns the antiemetic treatment, in controlled clinical trials many drugs have been shown to be effective and well tolerated in protecting against chemotherapy-induced emesis. The greater antiemetic efficacy of the new 5-HT_3 receptor antagonists, particularly against vomiting, is the most important result recently obtained in this field of scientific research. A regimen based on their combination with steroids is, however, almost always found superior [5-8]. About 9 years ago, the addition of corticosteroids to drug-blocking dopamine receptors (i.e., metoclopramide) led to the identification of the most efficacious treatment against cisplatin-induced emesis [9]. In designing (or in evaluating the results of) a clinical trial, it must be remembered that the efficacy of each agent can vary according to its dose, route and schedule of administration: these characteristics must be kept constant during the trial because they can partially explain the variability of the results obtained in different studies.

Factors Related to Chemotherapy

The antineoplastic chemotherapies differ in their emetogenic potential depending on the type of drugs used in the combination, their dosage and schedule, and the route of administration.

Every drug is currently classified according to its emetogenic potential as "high" (cisplatin, dacarbazine, mechlorethamine, dactinomycin), "moderate" (cyclophosphamide, cytosine arabinoside, anthracyclines, carboplatin, nitrosoureas, procarbazine), or "low" (methotrexate, mitomycin C, bleomycin, hydroxyurea, etoposide, fluorouracil, etc.) [1]. Although this rating reflects a real difference in the emetogenic potential based more on empirical clinical observations than on comparative studies, it is considered very important, so that the efficacy of antiemetic therapies is compared in patients submitted to chemotherapies belonging to only one of these three groups.

Generally, as the dose of a cytotoxic drug increases so does its emetogenic potential. Therefore, the doses are considered not only among the eligibility criteria (for instance, a patient receiving at least 50 mg/m^2 of cisplatin is eligible), but some subclasses of them can be used to define the levels of the prognostic factor "dose" in analysing the results (for example, patients receiving 90 mg/m^2 of cisplatin or less could be distinguished from those receiving larger doses).

Finally, as the infusion time of administration of the same dose increases, the incidence of nausea and vomiting generally decreases. This dependence, real or merely hypothetical, requires standardization of schedules.

Factors Related to the Patient Population

The variability of responses among patients and in the same patient in subsequent cycles of chemotherapy is well known. Many studies have been performed recently to identify the prognostic factors related to the patient population and to evaluate their importance. The main difficulty consists in taking into account the relationships among these factors and other variables, mainly those related to chemotherapy. For instance, the greater incidence of emesis observed among women could be due not only to their sex, but also to the type of chemotherapy (drugs and/or dose) most frequently most frequently used against cancers most common among women [10]. At any rate, even when adjusting for dose of chemotherapy, gender has often been found to significantly affect protection from and intensity of emesis [9,11,12].

Age of patients is another important variable in predicting the risk of nausea and vomiting: younger subjects are more susceptible to emesis than older ones. Age-related confounding factors which could affect the emetogenic potential, such as less aggressive chemotherapy, have been postulated but, even if adjusting for these, age may remain significant, allowing us to identify it as an independent prognostic factor [2].

A history of alcohol intake also seems to be an important prognostic factor: heavy drinkers are more protected against emesis than other patients [1].

The setting of administration of antineoplastic agents seems to play a role in determining the probability of emesis, particularly of nausea [13]: perhaps inpatients feel more protected by the environment than outpatients.

Finally, performance status, type of neoplasia, susceptibility to motion sickness, and emesis during pregnancy, although not often found important in explaining the variability of the response variables, could be considered in the analysis, after adjusting for the possible factors which could be confounders for them. When analysing data from a clinical trial, they are seldom found significant, probably because of a general homogeneity of the patient population with respect to them: only a meta-analysis based on more trials could allow detection of their effects on the response variables.

Study Population

The high variability of responses to antiemetic therapy and their sensitivity to changes in the pattern of prognostic factors induce us to adopt the broadest eligibility criteria to enroll patients in clinical trials. On the other hand, it is necessary that patients be sufficiently homogeneous with respect to some characteristics which could hinder unbiased comparisons, not only among the study groups but also between results of different studies. Particularly, the cycle and the emetogenic potential of chemotherapy should be chosen in advance so as to define the area under investigation.

Therefore, comparative studies should be carried out only in large patient populations in order to obtain results which are representative of a wide set of combinations of levels of prognostic factors: perhaps a cooperative (or multicentre) study among institutions that have interest and expertise in this particular field is the best solution. Efficient organisation, which allows centralized randomisation, careful design of the case record form, many meetings among the investigators, and an efficient system of monitoring, all assure good quality of the collected data.

Moreover, the sample size of an antiemetic trial is of critical importance: statistical tests must have sufficient power to detect the smallest clinically relevant difference. Although useful information can sometimes be obtained even from small studies, these results almost always necessitate validation by large, controlled studies, especially when the compared regimens differ markedly in efficacy or toxicity.

Finally, to avoid selection bias or other systematic errors, only consecutive cases should be considered and allocation of the patients to antiemetic treatments must be rigorously random, depending on the study design.

Study Design

When phase I-II studies of an antiemetic treatment have been completed, the activity of the agent must be compared to a standard regimen in a phase III randomised clinical trial.

Based on recent advances in this field, today the use of a placebo in the control group is considered as unethical [14], except in the case where an antiemetic regimen is not generally administered in clinical practice (for example, sometimes against delayed emesis) because of the lack of evidence of efficacy of some treatment. Any other experiment where the control group is not treated with the best known antiemetic therapy is also considered unethical. The association of a steroid with a 5-HT_3 receptor antagonist has been found the most efficacious antiemetic regimen against acute emesis induced by high-dose cisplatin. In spite of this, some papers showing results from clinical trials comparing treatments based only on 5-HT_3 receptor antagonists are still being accepted for publication [15,16].

A double-blind design is essential for obtaining unbiased estimations of efficacy, mostly because "soft responses", particularly those referring to protection from nausea and its severity, are evaluated in a clinical trial. Neither the investigator nor the patient should know the antiemetic regimen so as to eliminate any effect due to this expectation. However, effective blinding may sometimes be difficult to achieve. In our experience, the most practical way to assure blindness is to have only the research nurse, who is in charge of the randomisation, prepare and distribute the assigned treatments, while administration of drugs and evaluation of outcome is performed by other trained personnel [1].

Finally, two experimental designs, the parallel and crossover, are the most frequently used in antiemetic studies.

Completely Randomised Design

Homogeneity of the experimental groups with respect to the levels of the prognostic factors is achieved with random allocation of the patients to the antiemetic treatments. The different antiemetic efficacy of the regimens can thus be evaluated comparing a synthesis of the observed responses (i.e., means, percentages, and so on) from the experimental (parallel) groups during one or several cycles of chemotherapy.

Crossover Design

Each patient receives at each cycle of chemotherapy one of the different drugs being studied. Because of the brief time period between two subsequent cycles of chemotherapy, the condition of each patient can be hypothesized as being unmodified, in order to obtain responses under the same experimental conditions. Only the sequence of the treatments is randomised so as to avoid or reduce the effects related to the order in which the treatments are assigned.

One limitation of this experimental design is that it necessitates consideration of a number of cycles equal to (or multiple of) the number of treatments being studied.

Comparisons

At first analysis, two main advantages seem obvious in the preference of the crossover to the parallel design:
- it is a more powerful design (a smaller number of patients is required, given the fixed minimum difference of clinical importance, the level of significance and the power of the statistical test used to detect it);
- it offers the possibility to each patient to express a preference between the treatments.

However, its numerous disadvantages, listed below, lead us to prefer the completely randomised design:
i) emesis is a highly variable phenomenon; therefore, only a large patient population can offer a wide enough pattern of combination of levels of prognostic factors to allow us to consider the results obtained as reliable. In fact, when the experimental groups are small, the observed results can never be thought of as referring to a selected population, even if the eligibility and exclusion criteria are broad enough to assure a good representativity of the target population in the observed sample. If one treatment is found to be more efficacious than another, does its superiority apply to all patients or only to those similar to those observed?
ii) the crossover design does not allow evaluation of the persistence of antiemetic activity in subsequent cycles of chemotherapy;
iii) the crossover design cannot be considered as reliable when a large number of patients have been lost from one cycle of chemotherapy to the following. In our experience, 20-30% of patients were lost from one cycle of cisplatin chemotherapy to the next. Because it is impossible to consider the lost patients as a random sample, this could lead us to think of a selection bias in evaluating the responses;
iv) another serious bias could arise if the patient's condition does not remain the same from one cycle of chemotherapy to the following.

Therefore, we think that the results obtained by a crossover study should be validated by a larger, completely randomised study. The exception to this would be a sufficiently large parallel study at the first cycle of chemotherapy, where a crossover was planned at the second cycle, mainly to test patient preference for one treatment or the other.

Efficacy Evaluation

Clinical trials comparing the antiemetic efficacy of two or more regimens are characterized by a short follow-up, at most a few days after each cycle of chemotherapy. Moreover, because of their ease of management, mistakes in enrolment or randomisation of patients seldom occur. Therefore, there are generally small differences between the patient population evaluable according to the "intention-to-treat" principle and that evaluable for clinical efficacy.

The aim of this section is to discuss some methodological topics and to outline statistical methods which should be used in analysing the results.

Unifactorial Analysis of Acute Emesis

If randomisation has allowed us to have similar arms with respect to the levels of prognostic factors, the most important results can be obtained from a unifactorial analysis comparing a synthesis of the individual responses (means, percentages, and so on) between the experimental groups (defined by the antiemetic treatments).

Because of the type of response, non-parametric tests must be preferred. Generally, their asymptotic approximations can be successfully used because the experimental groups are large.

Obviously, if a parallel design is chosen, tests for independent samples must be used:
chi-square test for dichotomic responses, Mann-Whitney U-test or Kruskall-Wallis test if, respectively, two or more means are to be compared, and so on.

When comparing two proportions, a 95% confidence interval for their difference can give useful information.

A unifactorial analysis for each prognostic factor should also be performed, although its conclusions should be interpreted cautiously because of the correlations among them: only the subsequent multifactorial analysis will give reliable results.

If the trial is based on a crossover design analysing clinical efficacy, non-parametric tests for paired data should generally be performed (i.e., Mc Nemar's test or Wilcoxon's matched-pairs signed-ranks test, when comparing, respectively, two proportions or two means). But even if randomisation of the sequences of treatments yields a good balance between groups with respect to prognostic factors, the existence of possible cycle and period effects should be investigated, possibly using multifactorial models which allow evaluation of the efficacy adjusting for these effects. Finally, the analysis of patient preference for one or the other antiemetic regimen has to be carried out using specific tests, like Prescott's test [17], designed to evaluate the indifference, i.e., the lack of a choice in favour of either of the treatments.

Multifactorial Analysis of Acute Emesis at First Cycle of Chemotherapy

Even when there is a good balance of the prognostic factors among the experimental groups, it is our opinion that a multifactorial analysis should be performed. Its aim is essentially to identify the prognostic factors which influence the response variable, adjusting for the other factors and for treatment, and to find if there exists some subgroup of patients where the antiemetic treatments have a different behaviour from that observed in the whole group. This latter aim can be achieved by examining the significance of the two-order (or higher) interaction contrasts, where one factor is the treatment.

The clinical importance of these findings is evident.

First of all, appropriate utilization of the knowledge that the prognostic factors can significantly influence the responses allows us to obtain a more precise estimate of the incidence of nausea and vomiting in patients treated with a particular antiemetic regimen. An example of this type of analysis, performed in a large number of cisplatin-treated patients receiving two antiemetic combinations (ondansetron + dexamethasone (OND + DEX) and metoclopramide + dexamethasone + diphenhydramine (MTC + DEX + DIP)) has been reported [13].

Secondly, the identification of subsets of patients where the outcomes were found to be different from those observed in the whole group (i.e., the differences between treatments were strongly decreased, or increased, with respect to those detected in the whole group) allows us to adopt more specific clinical decisions for each subgroup, also on the basis of the different tolerability and cost of the treatments. This could subsequently modify clinical practice or, at least, suggest some hypotheses to be submitted to a future trial. Unfortunately, significant results can never be reached because of the small dimensions of the subgroups where the statistical analysis is performed. Under well defined conditions (i.e., all trials were conducted with the same methodology and all data were available), however, the hypotheses suggested by a subgroup analysis could become the main purpose of a meta-analysis.

Thirdly, an analysis of the significant prognostic factors is an essential part of the evaluation of the results of all studies on antiemetic treatments. Its omission makes the interpretation of the results difficult and may lead to inappropriate conclusions. Moreover, knowledge of their importance allows correct planning of any further clinical study on antiemetic therapy.

There are many statistical models that can be used to perform a multifactorial analysis; the choice mainly depends on the type of response variable. In fact, if the response variable is dichotomic, logistic models should be used, while if it is a count (i.e., number of emetic episodes), log-linear models should be used. As an example of the use of the results obtained with a multifactorial analysis for acute cisplatin-induced emesis at first cycle of chemotherapy, let us consider the logistic model for the probability of vomiting which identified 'Treatment' (A = ondansetron + dexamethasone (OND + DEX); B = metoclopramide + dexamethasone + diphenhydramine (MTC + DEX + DIP)), 'Dose of cisplatin' (H = ≥90 mg/m^2, L = <90 mg/m^2), and 'Sex' (M = male, F = female) as significant factors [13].

Main effects and interactions	z-test	P<	parameter estimation
General mean	-6.02	0.001	-2.808
Treatment (B - A)	3.77	0.001	1.654
Dose of cisplatin (H - L)	3.79	0.001	1.916
Sex (F - M)	2.83	0.003	0.983
Treatment x Dose (B-A)(H-L)	-2.21	0.014	-1.283

Regarding the main effects, treatment A is more efficacious than B (the sign of the significant contrast between treatments is positive: the probability of vomiting is greater among the patients who received B than among those who were treated with A); a high dose of cisplatin increases the probability of vomiting, and females are less protected than males. The interaction gives useful information: the superiority of A with respect to B is higher in patients who received low doses (the sign of the interaction is negative).

The model allows us to identify 8 subgroups of patients for each of which it is easy to calculate the correspondent probability of vomiting, using the parameter estimations. For instance, let us estimate the probability of vomiting for a female (F), treated with a low dose of cisplatin (L), who received the OND + DEX combination (A).

The estimated linear predictor is:

$$LP = \text{mean} + \text{treatment} + \text{dose} + \text{sex} + \text{interaction} = -2.808 + 1.654x1 + 1.916x0 + 0.983x1 - 1.283x0 = -0.171$$

and, therefore, the correspondent probability is

$$P = \exp(LP) / [1 + \exp(LP)] = 0.457.$$

For each of the 8 subgroups of patients, defined by levels of significant factors, the correspondent probability can be calculated: it is a useful tool for clinical decisions.

Multifactorial Analysis of Acute Emesis in Subsequent Cycles of Chemotherapy

When analysing data from subsequent cycles of chemotherapy, two independent main topics should be highlighted: the importance of the dependence effect on the results observed at previous cycles and the persistence effect of each treatment.

Both these phenomena can be analysed only in the group of patients who underwent all considered cycles of chemotherapy, excluding the subjects lost from each cycle to the subsequent one. But this selection of patients can never be regarded as a random occurrence and if this hypothesis is verified (it is sufficient to observe in detail the causes of patient loss) standard statistical analysis would be affected by selection bias and the results must be interpreted with great caution. Conversely, if it is possible to show that the loss of patients from one cycle of chemotherapy to the subsequent one is not relevant (i.e., less than 15%) or the causes are not related to the scant antiemetic efficacy of therapies, then it is very interesting to analyse both the dependence effect and the persistence of antiemetic efficacy of each therapy.

Many studies have shown that the dependence effect is the main prognostic factor [12, 13]: patients who were protected against emesis at first cycle have an inferior probability of emesis at the subsequent one, while those who had emesis are at high risk to experience it again. This confirms that the probability of emesis mainly depends on the patient's characteristics, i.e., on his personal attitude to emesis.

From a statistical point of view, when considering complete protection or not as the response, it is easy to introduce the dependence effect as an explicative variable, both in the parallel [18] and crossover design [19], using logistic linear models or, equivalently, log-linear models.

Only by adjusting for this important prognostic factor can the effect of the treatment be correctly evaluated; without considering it, the superiority of a treatment at a subsequent cycle could be due only to its greater efficacy in previous cycles. For instance, let us consider the evaluation of the difference between two antiemetic treatments (A and B) in terms of complete protection from vomiting, at the second cycle of chemotherapy. On unifactorial analysis A is found significantly superior to B. This can be due either to a real superiority of A at the second cycle, or to the greater efficacy of A at the first cycle alone, as A has the same efficacy as B at the second cycle. Protecting more patients at the first cycle because of the lesser probability of emesis of the patients who did not vomit, A is again found more efficacious than B at the second cycle. To detect what is the model which has generated the data, it is sufficient to evaluate at second cycle the effect of the treatment, adjusting for the dependence effect. If the treatment is found significant, we can infer the greater efficacy of A also at the second cycle; conversely, if, when adjusting for the dependence effect, treatment A is not found to be significantly more efficacious than

Main effects	z-test	P<	Parameter estimation
General mean	-2.39	0.017	-0.599
Dependence effect (D_{12})	5.56	0.001	0.967
Treatment (B - A)	1.99	0.047	0.661

B, its superiority could be attributable only to its greater efficacy at the first cycle (and, therefore, to the effect of the dependence).

As an example of how to interpret and use the results of a multifactorial analysis of acute emesis at the second cycle, let us consider the corresponding logistic model for the probability of vomiting shown in the aforementioned study (see schedule above).

Although the dependence effect is the most important factor to explain the variability of probability of acute vomiting at the second cycle, the effect of the treatment, even when adjusting for dependence, remains significant: OND + DEX (treatment A) gives greater protection from acute emesis not only for its superiority shown at the first cycle, but also because of its greater efficacy at the second cycle. These two significant factors allow us to identify 4 subgroups of patients for each of which it is possible to estimate the probability of vomiting during the first 24 hours after chemotherapy. Let us consider a patient treated with B (MTC+DEX+DIP) who did not vomit at the first cycle. The linear predictor estimate is:

$LP = - 0.599 + 0.967x0 + 0.661x1 = 0.062.$

Therefore, the correspondent probability is

$P = \exp(0.062) / [1 + \exp(0.062)] = 0.515.$

If, on the other hand, the patient did vomit at the first cycle, his probability of also vomiting at the second is:

$LP = - 0.599 + 0.967x1 + 0.661x1 = 1.029; P = 0.736.$

Emesis at the first cycle produces an increase of more than 22% in the probability of vomiting at the second cycle.

Now, let us consider the patients who received OND + DEX (treatment A). If they vomited at the first cycle, their probability of also vomiting at the second is:

$LP = - 0.599 + 0.967x1 + 0.661x0 = 0.368; P = 0.597.$

If, on the other hand, they were protected against vomiting at the first cycle, the correspondent probability is:

$LP = - 0.599; P = 0.354.$

Nevertheless, while the persistence of the antiemetic efficacy of a treatment can be considered as being conceptually independent of the dependence effect, from a methodological point of view the former is also involved in the selection bias phenomenon.

In fact, antiemetic therapies sometimes tend to lose their efficacy in subsequent cycles of chemotherapy [12]. If the selection of patients from one cycle to the next is mainly due to reasons other than the non-efficacy of the antiemetic regimen, considering only the patients who underwent all cycles of chemotherapy, it is possible to evaluate the persistence of efficacy of each treatment by using simple statistical tests, such as Wilcoxon's signed-ranks matched-pairs test, if the number of cycles is equal to two, or Cochran's Q-test, when it is greater than two.

But, when the loss of patients from one cycle to the next is mainly due to low antiemetic efficacy of a treatment, the presence of a selection bias can be suspected. It might happen that the treatment which was found inferior at the first cycle proves to be the most efficacious at the second. This fact may be explained in terms of selection bias. The less efficacious treatment, not protecting many patients at first cycle against emesis, can produce their withdrawal; therefore, the patients treated with it who will undergo the second cycle have a worse intrinsic attitude to emesis. Instead, the most efficacious therapy has protected more patients at the first cycle, including those with an intrinsic high risk of emesis. At the second cycle, the presence of these latter, who have a greater probability of emesis, can produce an apparently worse performance of the treatment which in actual fact is the most efficacious.

In conclusion, great care must be taken in analysing the entity and the causes of patient selection from one cycle to the following, keeping in mind that if one of the main causes of this loss is the scant efficacy of a treatment, the results of the statistical analysis must be interpreted very cautiously. In fact, this selection bias seems to be unfavourable to the most efficacious antiemetic regimen and, therefore, when performing a statistical analysis without considering the causes of the withdrawals from each cycle to the subsequent one, the superior antiemetic regimen could be erroneously found to be that which has less persistence in efficacy.
These considerations can also affect the choice of a crossover design. In fact, its results can be referred mainly to patients who were more protected against emesis at first cycle and not to the patient population defined by the eligibility and exclusion criteria.

On the Relationship Between Nausea and Vomiting

As is highlighted above, at each cycle of chemotherapy complete protection from nausea and vomiting are almost always separately analysed, despite their strong correlation. But, as is well known, this relationship can hide a confounding effect or an interaction between these phenomena. More clearly, if treatment A is found superior to treatment B against both nausea and vomiting, one of the following mutually exclusive events can be considered [20]:
a) A is really more efficacious than B in preventing nausea and vomiting;
b) Confounding. The presence/absence of vomiting (nausea) is a confounding factor for the different efficacy of A and B in complete protection from nausea (vomiting); A is superior to B only in preventing vomiting (nausea), but has the same efficacy as B in the prevention of nausea (vomiting);
c) Interaction. Let us consider protection from vomiting as the dependent variable; the same consideration can be made for complete protection from nausea.
A is superior to B in preventing vomiting only in the subset of patients who had nausea; in the other group (i.e., patients who did not suffer from nausea) B was found more (or equally) efficacious than A;
d) Correlation effect. Both confounding factors (b) are present: A and B have the same efficacy in preventing both nausea and vomiting (the superiority of A in protecting against nausea and vomiting is not real).
Recently, a new method for analysing data in the presence of a pair of dichotomic responses has been proposed [20]. Let us fit two logistic models, assuming as dependent variables in the first model complete protection from vomiting and in the second complete protection from nausea, and as factors the treatment and the response variable which was not considered as dependent. If the interaction term is not found significant, (c) can be excluded and, therefore, additive models allow us to investigate which structure among (a), (b) and (d) can have produced the observed data. More precisely, when performing additive models,
- the superiority of A is due to a pure correlation effect (d) if, after adjusting for the other response variable, the effect of the treatment is not found significant, neither for complete protection from vomiting nor for complete protection from nausea;
- A is really superior to B against both vomiting and nausea if, after adjusting for the other response variable, A is again found significantly more efficacious than B against vomiting as well as against nausea (a);
- the superiority of A against nausea (vomiting) is due only to a confounding effect (b); A is more efficacious than B only against vomiting (nausea) if, adjusting for nausea (vomiting), A is again found significantly superior to B, but, adjusting for vomiting (nausea), A and B are not found significantly different with respect to complete protection from nausea (vomiting).
The presence of a confounding effect has often been found when data from recent trials were re-analysed. Therefore, an investigation of the effects of the correlation of the two responses should always be carried out in a separate analysis.

For example, on re-analysing data from the aforementioned study [13], at the first cycle of chemotherapy OND + DEX were found significantly more efficacious than MTC + DEX + DIP against both nausea and vomiting:

Complete protection from vomiting (nausea)	OND + DEX	MTC + DEX + DIP
YES	107 (105)	78 (86)
NO	29 (31)	53 (45)
no. of patients	136	131

A strong correlation between complete protection from vomiting and nausea was observed, however, the relative risk to have nausea, given the presence/absence of vomiting, was equal to 4.61.
In both logistic models the interaction term was not found significant; this allowed us to consider only the additive models.
In the first model (dependent variable: presence/absence of vomiting; factors: presence/absence of nausea, treatment), even when adjusting for the presence/absence of nausea, the treatment effect remains significant: OND + DEX is really superior to MTC + DEX + DIP against vomiting. In fact, complete protection from vomiting obtained by OND+DEX/MTC+DEX+DIP was:
- in patients who had nausea: 41.9% / 26.7%;
- in patients who did not have nausea: 89.5% / 76.7%.

In the second logistic model (dependent variable: presence/absence of nausea; factors: presence/absence of vomiting, treatment), with adjusting for the presence/absence of vomiting, the treatments were not found significantly different. In spite of the results obtained at unifactorial analysis, they have the same efficacy against nausea; i.e., presence/absence of vomiting is a confounding factor for the different efficacy of the treatments on complete protection from nausea. In fact, even when considering the raw data, the percentages of patients protected from nausea receiving OND+DEX / MTC+DEX+DIP, were:
- in patients who vomited: 37.9% / 37.7%;
- in patients who did not vomit: 87.9% / 84.6%.

The significantly greater efficacy of OND+DEX in preventing nausea, detected at unifactorial analysis, can be attributed only to its superiority in the control of vomiting and, therefore, in preventing any concomitant nausea. These results suggest the existence of at least two kinds of nausea, the first independent of vomiting (against which the two regimens can be considered as having the same efficacy), and the second concomitant to it (the kind of nausea generated by the same mechanism which produces vomiting).

Analysis of Delayed Emesis

Delayed emesis should be analysed considering both the day-by-day responses and those for the whole period, generally from days 2-4 or 2-5 because of the decrease in frequency and severity of emesis in subsequent days, although some authors have recently tried to obtain synthetic information also from day 6 to the next cycle of chemotherapy. Another way to evaluate delayed emesis is to consider the worst day, i.e., the day among the second and the fifth when the worst emesis was observed. Whichever evaluation is used, analysis of delayed emesis should be carried out considering its dependence on acute emesis observed during the same cycle of chemotherapy (and, possibly, on both acute and delayed emesis at previous cycles). As has been widely demonstrated [21], patients who were protected against acute emesis have a lesser probability of delayed emesis and, therefore, the superiority of treatment A with respect to treatment B could be due only to the greater protection obtained during the first 24 hours. The methodology of the analysis of such a dependence effect has been described earlier in this chapter, without considering the selection bias, which is generally absent as only few patients are evaluable for acute but not for delayed emesis. In early studies, when really efficacious therapies were not yet available, delayed emesis did not receive great attention because of its less severe nature with respect to acute emesis. Perhaps this is the main reason for the lack of experimental studies on the efficacy of regimens against delayed emesis. At present, given the good control of acute emesis obtained by the combination of steroids with 5-HT_3 receptor antagonists, specific trials on delayed emesis should be carried out in patients receiving either highly or moderately emetogenic chemotherapy. Based on the most efficacious antiemetic therapies against acute emesis, patients should be randomised to receive a treatment specifically designed against delayed emesis, chosen on the basis of ethical, methodological and economic considerations.

Tolerability

Today, the most frequent adverse events which can arise during clinical trials on antiemetic efficacy of therapeutic regimens are sufficiently known. Simple statistical tests for comparing proportions, which base their logical foundations on randomisation, are sufficient to investigate the different incidence of each event among the experimental groups.
A substantial improvement in the knowledge of this issue can be obtained only by meta-analysis conducted in a very large patient population so as to make evident the incidence of rare events. Obviously, such a meta-analysis should be founded on studies which adopted a similar protocol; therefore, international standardisation of the methodologies and true availability of data are strongly recommended.

Conclusions

In the last few years, a substantial improvement has been made in the control of chemotherapy-induced emesis and in the understanding of the great variability of this phenomenon among subjects. There has been the discovery of the antiemetic properties of the 5-HT_3 receptor antagonists, which, in combination with steroids, are to be regarded as the most powerful antiemetic regimen. Moreover, large comparative trials have been carried out in which better measurement tools were used and the results analysed with more sophisticated statistical methodologies. This has allowed us to highlight the importance of the prognostic factors connected with the individual patient's characteristics. Particularly, the relevance of the dependence effect of a response variable on previously observed results has been correctly evaluated.
As is well known, however, the costs of the 5-HT_3 receptor antagonists are greatly superior to those of the previous standard antiemetic therapies, which were essentially based on antidopaminergic drugs. When a trial on the antiemetic efficacy of several regimens is conducted, a concomitant pharmacoeconomic study should therefore be carried out to obtain information about the treatments in terms of cost/efficacy.
As a future perspective, new knowledge in some fields not yet sufficiently investigated is to be expected, particularly regarding delayed emesis, the comparative efficacy of different 5-HT_3 receptor antagonists, and their optimal dose. Moreover, because of the dependence effect, patients who suffered from emesis at the first cycle of chemotherapy (especially if they had 3 or more vomiting episodes) have a great probability of vomiting again in subsequent cycles: as the therapies usually employed in clinical practice are insufficient for these patients, new regimens should be designed and subsequently submitted to clinical trials.
Research into antiemetics has developed to such a degree that we believe the organisation of a Consensus Conference, including the following aims, would be of great usefulness.

a) To standardize the methodological issues of clinical trials.
Based on a list of the most widely accepted prognostic factors that are to be investigated, it is possible to define a Case Record Form that could be used in any trial, obviously leaving each investigator free to add any other item he considers useful in his own study. Also, by standardizing the dose, schedule and route of administration of both chemotherapy and antiemetic prophylaxis as well as any other setting modalities, more comparable data among studies would be obtained. In this way it becomes possible to perform a meta-analysis on the largest patient population and analyse more precisely the importance of the prognostic factors as well as detect rare adverse events. Moreover, in evaluating responses, the cutoff separating acute from delayed emesis should be accurately defined: can it still be maintained at 24 hours from the administration of chemotherapy or should it be modified because of the increase in the time to onset of emesis thanks to new 5-HT_3 receptor antagonists?

b) To define ethical aspects of clinical trials on

the antiemetic efficacy of therapies.
Unethical trials are sometimes carried out. For instance, it is not infrequent that in a trial the experimental treatment consists of 5-HT_3 receptor antagonists alone, without the addition of a steroid, while it is proven that only their combination can be considered as the most efficacious antiemetic regimen.

c) To strongly insist that the data collected by pharmaceutical companies be made available to researchers.
In this way many interesting epidemiological studies could be carried out which could substantially increase our knowledge of this important field of scientific research in clinical oncology.

REFERENCES

1 Tonato M, Roila F, Del Favero A: Methodology of antiemetic trials: a review. Ann Oncol 1991 (2): 107-114
2 Del Favero A, Roila F, Basurto C et al: Assessment of nausea. Eur J Clin Pharmacol 1991 (38):115-120
3 Chevallier B, on behalf of the Granisetron Study Group: The control of acute cisplatin-induced emesis. A comparative study of granisetron and a combination regimen of high-dose metoclopramide and dexamethasone. Br J Cancer 1993 (68):176-180
4 Soukop M on behalf of the Granisetron Study Group: A dose-finding study of granisetron, a novel antiemetic, in patients receiving high-dose cisplatin. Support Care Cancer 1994 (2):177-183
5 Roila F, Tonato M, Cognetti F et al: Prevention of cisplatin-induced emesis: a double-blind multicenter randomized crossover study comparing ondansetron and ondansetron plus dexamethasone. J Clin Oncol 1991 (9):675-678
6 Smyth F, Coleran RE, Nicholson M et al: Does dexamethasone enhance control of acute cispaltin induced emesis by ondansetron? Br Med J 1991 (303):1423-1426
7 Hesketh P, Harvey WH, Harker WG et al: A randomized, double-blind comparison of intravenous ondansetron alone and in combination with intravenous dexamethasone in the prevention of high-dose cisplatin-induced emesis. J Clin Oncol 1994 (12):596-600
8 Italian Group for Antiemetic Research: Dexamethasone, granisetron, or both for the prevention of nausea and vomiting during chemotherapy for cancer. N Engl J Med 1995 (322):1-5
9 Roila F, Tonato M, Basurto C et al: Antiemetic activity of high doses of metoclopramide combined with methylprednisolone vs metoclopramide alone in cisplatin-treated cancer patients: a randomized double-blind trial of the Italian Oncology Group for Clinical Research. J Clin Oncol 1987 (5):141-149
10 Pater J, Slamet L, Zee B, Osoba D, Warr D, Rusthoven J: Inconsistency of prognostic factors for both chemotherapy-nausea and vomiting. Support Care Cancer 1994 (2):161-166
11 Roila F, Tonato M, Basurto C et al: Antiemetic activity of two different high doses of metoclopramide in cisplatin-treated cancer patients: a randomized double-blind trial of the Italian Oncology Group for Clinical Research. Cancer Treat Rep 1985 (69): 1353-1357
12 Roila F, Tonato M, Basurto C et al: Protection from nausea and vomiting in cisplatin-treated patients: high-dose metoclopramide combined with methylprednisolone versus metoclopramide combined with dexamethasone and diphenhydramine: a study of the Italian Oncology Group for Clinical Research. J Clin Oncol 1989 (7):1693-1700
13 Italian Group for Antiemetic Research: Difference in persistence of two antiemetic regimens on acute emesis during cisplatin chemotherapy. J Clin Oncol 1993 (11):2396-2404
14 Roila F, Tonato M, Del Favero A: Publication of unethical studies on the treatment of chemotherapy-induced emesis (letter to Editor). J Clin Oncol 1991 (9):891-892
15 Ruff P, Paska W, Goedhals L et al on behalf of the Ondansetron and Granisetron Emesis Study Group: Ondansetron compared with granisetron in the prophylaxis of cisplatin induced acute emesis: a multicenter double-blind, randomized, parallel-group study. Oncology 1994 (51):113-118
16 Sorbe BG, Hogberg T, Glimelius B et al: A randomized, multicenter study comparing the efficacy and tolerability of tropisetron, a new 5-HT_3 receptor antagonist, with a metoclopramide-containing antiemetic cocktail in the prevention of cisplatin-induced emesis. Cancer 1994 (73):445-454
17 Prescott RJ: The comparison of success rates in cross-over trials in the presence of an order effect. Appl Statistics 1981 (30):9-15
18 Ballatori E: Modelli logistici nell'analisi di dati binari con misure ripetute. Proceedings of the 'II Congresso Nazionale dell'Associazione Italiana di Statistica Medica e Programmazione Socio Sanitaria', Pavia, 26-28 Oct 1989:271-278
19 Kenward MG and Jones B: A log-linear model for binary cross-over data. Appl Statistics 1987 (36): 192-204
20 Italian Group for Antiemetic Research: On the relationship between nausea and vomiting in patients undergoing chemotherapy. Support Care Cancer 1994 (2):171-176
21 Italian Group for Antiemetic Research: Cisplatin-induced delayed emesis: pattern and prognostic factors during three subsequent cycles. Ann Oncol 1994 (5):585-589

Prevention of Acute Cisplatin-Induced Nausea and Vomiting

Pieter H.M. De Mulder [1] and Jaap Verweij [2]

1 Department of Internal Medicine, Division of Medical Oncology, University Hospital Nijmegen, Geert Grooteplein 8, 6500 HB Nijmegen, The Netherlands
2 Department of Medical Oncology, Rotterdam Cancer Institute/Daniel den Hoed Cancer Centre, Groene Hilledijk 301, 3075 EA Rotterdam, The Netherlands

All cytotoxic drugs can induce nausea and vomiting depending on the type of agent, dose, route and schedule of administration [1]. This variability underlines the differences in mechanisms responsible for the difference in onset and duration of this side-effect. Cisplatin is one of the most widely used cytotoxic agents and has significantly contributed to the curative potential of chemotherapy. However, the spectrum of side-effects is substantial and its capacity to induce nausea and vomiting is unprecedented. High doses of cisplatin produce acute nausea and vomiting in almost all patients unless antiemetic drugs are used. Therefore much effort has been made to control this distressing side-effect and the present status will be updated in this chapter. This overview is restricted to control of acute nausea and vomiting, arbitrarily defined as occurring in the first 24 hours after the start of treatment. The onset is generally within the first 4 hours, reaching a peak intensity between 4 and 10 hours after drug administration. The important role of cisplatin in the delayed phase will be reviewed elsewhere in this volume.

The mechanisms involved in cisplatin-induced acute emesis have been studied both *in vitro* and in animal models. Three possible pathways can be discerned: 1) a direct release of 5-hydroxytryptamine (5-HT) due to damage of the enterochromaffin cells in the mucosa of the upper gastrointestinal tract [2]; 2) alterations of gastrointestinal motility [3]; 3) an indirect release of 5-HT by activation of enteric cholinergic neurones [4]. The antiemetic drugs currently in use for the prevention of cisplatin-induced emesis all have their influence on one or more of these pathways, sometimes at different sites of the arch.

Role of Dopamine Antagonists as Single Agents and in Combinations

This group of compounds comprises the phenothiazines, the butyrophenones, the benzamide derivative alizapride and the procainamide derivative metoclopramide (MCP) [1]. Within this group MCP is the drug of choice for the prevention of cisplatin-induced emesis. Until recently MCP was thought to mediate its antiemetic effect mainly by a blockade of the peripheral dopamine D_2 receptors and those in the chemoreceptor trigger zone. However, it has now been demonstrated that at higher doses MCP also shows affinity with the 5-HT_3 receptor, leading to a blockade of signal transduction via this receptor [5].

At conventional doses (0.15-0.3 mg/kg) only limited antiemetic activity is obtained. However, higher dosages were found to be much more effective [6]. This initial breakthrough has later been confirmed in many investigations and has led to a further refinement of the dose, schedule and co-medication.

In randomised studies, high-dose MCP given as a repeated intravenous infusion was superior to prochlorperazine, 9-tetrahydrocannabinol, butyrophenones, alizapride and dexamethasone in the control of acute cisplatin-induced emesis [6-12]. The efficacy of MCP has been correlated with the attainment of high serum levels (>850 ng/ml) [13] and the maintenance of steady-state levels [14]. In other studies different pharmacokinetic analyses failed to establish a clear relationship between MCP levels and outcome [15,16]. One of the reasons might be that the main mechanism of action is the interaction with both the dopamine

D_2 and 5-HT_3 receptor in a competitive manner, requiring a certain dose at a certain moment. Receptor affinity and kinetics are probably more relevant when at least a threshold amount of drug is available. The clinical observations seem to support this hypothesis because a great number of different MCP schedules do not really show significantly different results. When a single dose of 4-6 mg/kg was compared with two times 3 mg/kg in combination with the same dosages of dexamethasone and lorazepam, a similar overall complete response rate of 60% was found [17,18]. The efficacy of MCP when given as 1 mg/kg bolus followed by 0.5 mg/kg/h for 24 hours was superior to 1 mg/kg i.v. bolus every 2 hours 5 or 6 times in a few relatively small studies [19-22]. In one study where MCP was given with lorazepam, dexamethasone and diphenhydramine [22] (unblinded, crossover in 58 evaluable patients), total control of nausea and vomiting was 65% versus 90% in favour of the continuous infusion arm. The design of this study is not optimal because of the unblinded nature. Of practical importance is that MCP and cisplatin could be given through the same line, a disadvantage is that this approach is only feasible when cisplatin is given on an inpatient basis. Another route of administration is oral MCP (2-3 mg/kg) with related sufficient serum levels and adequate antiemetic control in patients receiving cisplatin 60 mg/m² [23,24].

It is generally accepted that combination therapy is the treatment of choice when intermediate or high-dose cisplatin is given and high-dose MCP is the backbone of the antiemetic regimen. All studies combining corticosteroids with MCP have shown either superiority or equivalence, with patient's preference for the combination arm [17,25-28]. The two most frequently used compounds are dexamethasone and methylprednisolone. There is no consensus regarding the optimal dose and schedule of corticosteroids. Dose ranges used were 250-1000 mg for methylprednisolone and 8-50 mg for dexamethasone [1]. There is no proven advantage for high-dose or more frequent administration (i.e., once or more) [29]. The potential value of adding benzodiazepines because of their anxiolytic, sedative and minimal antiemetic properties, has been extensively investigated [17,27,29,30]. In a randomised study lorazepam showed better control of acute cisplatin-induced emesis compared to methylprednisolone [29]. In combination with prochlorperazine, dexamethasone or MCP, an improved control of acute induced emesis was seen [27,31,32]. Addition of lorazepam to the combination dexamethasone and MCP did not result in an improved efficacy but akathisia (restlessness) and anxiety were observed less frequently [17]. The sedation allowed the inpatient to sleep well and the overall appreciation of this combination was reflected in a significant patient preference for the lorazepam combination [17]. Interesting is the fact that there was no correlation between the degree of sedation and the antiemetic effect, which suggests an additive mechanism of action. The reduction of akathisia has led to the omission of standard diphenhydramine in combinations were lorazepam is added to MCP.

In Table 1 the recommendations for optimal use of MCP in combinations are given.

The toxicity of MCP, especially when used at the appropriate dose, is caused by the dopamine antagonistic effects of this compound. Side-effects comprise mild sedation, diarrhoea, akathisia and extrapyramidal reactions [1]. The incidence of extrapyramidal reactions is not only dependent on the dose but also on the route of administration and the age of the patients. Patients less than 30 years of age revealed an incidence of 27% in contrast with those over 30 years where an incidence of 2% was observed. There is no explanation for this

Table 1. Different MCP containing regimens for cisplatin-induced emesis

Cisplatin dose	Antiemetics*	Frequency/day
≥100 mg/m²	MCP 2-3 mg/kg iv	2-3 x
	+ lorazepam 1.5 mg/m²	1 x
	+ dexamethasone 10-20 mg	1 x
40-80 mg/m²	MCP 2-3 mg/kg i.v.	2-3 x
	+ lorazepam 1 mg/m² or	1 x
	diphenhydramine 50-100 mg **	1 x
	+ dexamethasone 10-20 mg	1x
<40 mg/m²	MCP 1-2 mg/kg	2-3 x
	+ lorazepam 1mg/m²	1 x
	diphenhydramine 50-100 mg **	1 x
	± dexamethasone 10-20 mg	1 x

* Instead of dexamethasone methylprednisolone 250-500 mg i.v. can be used

** An alternative is piperidene 2-5 mg i.v.

finding but it is the main reason why MCP is rarely used in children treated with high-dose cisplatin. After oral medication the incidence of acute dystonic reactions in both categories was clearly enhanced, with an incidence of 75% and 8%, respectively [23]. The abovementioned side-effects can be ameliorated with antihistamines or benzodiazepines (see Table 1). Corticosteroids have been shown to reduce the incidence of diarrhoea [33].

5-Hydroxytryptamine (5-HT_3) Antagonists

The development of compounds with a highly specific affinity for the 5-HT_3 receptor and the recognition that high-dose MCP may exert its activity mainly through the blockade of this receptor has marked the start of a new era in the treatment of chemotherapy-induced acute nausea and vomiting. The 5-HT_3 receptor is involved, besides its other functions, in the mediation of nausea/vomiting and gastrointestinal motility. At present most data support a predominant role of the receptors present on the vagal afferent neurones located in the upper gut.

Ondansetron, granisetron and tropisetron are the most widely studied representatives of this new class of antiemetics. They display marked differences with respect to their structure, receptor affinity, selectivity, metabolism, dose response, duration of action and potency (µg/kg drug required to protect 50% of the animals after a standard stimulus) in preclinical models [34-38]. There is no definite proof at the moment that such differences are relevant from a clinical point of view. The clinical role of these 3 compounds will be discussed below.

Ondansetron, Efficacy in Single-Day Cisplatin Regimens

At present most of the published clinical experience with 5-HT_3 antagonists has been with ondansetron. The development of this compound has been different in Europe and the USA, which is a disadvantage. The first studies in Europe investigated different dose levels with an intermittent schedule where ondansetron was diluted in 100 ml of normal saline and given intravenously over 15 minutes 30 minutes prior to the start of cisplatin administration [39,40]. Based on the information that a consistent dose of 30 ng/ml would block all 5-HT_3 receptors and the knowledge that this could be achieved with a bolus dose of 8 mg followed by 24 mg given as a continuous infusion over 24 hours, this regimen was selected for the subsequent randomised studies in Europe. Two double-blind, randomised, crossover studies showed a significant advantage in favour of ondansetron both for vomiting and nausea in comparison with MCP given as a loading dose of 3 mg/kg followed by 4 mg/kg over 8 hours [40,41]. No episodes of emesis or only one or two were seen in 75% [40] and 72% [41] of the ondansetron-treated patients and 42% and 41%, respectively, of those who received MCP. The regimen of both ondansetron and MCP was different from the one most frequently used in the USA. Furthermore, the potential for a treatment by period interaction is one of the disadvantages of the crossover design, although no such interaction was observed in these studies.

In the USA 3-to-6-times-daily bolus doses of ondansetron (0.01-0.48 mg/kg) at 2-8 hour intervals were evaluated. Below 0.1 mg/kg antiemetic responses were poor and best responses were seen at a level of 0.12-0.18 mg/kg without further improvement at higher doses [42-46]. The dose of 0.15 mg/kg x 3 (q 3-4 hours) resulted in a complete control in 40-45% of the chemotherapy-naive patients in the first 24 hours and was selected for comparative studies. In a single-blind study this regimen was compared with MCP (2 mg/kg i.v. x 6) in 307 patients treated with high-dose (≥ 100 mg/m^2) cisplatin [47]. With ondansetron a complete protection was seen in 40% of the patients versus 30% with MCP. In view of these results the dose schedule seemed not very critical. This can be explained partly by the fact that during MCP treatment the peak incidence of vomiting was seen in the first 6-12 hours [42,43], which suggests that this is the period with the strongest emetogenic stimulus after cisplatin. This period corresponds with an increased urinary excretion of 5-hydroxyindole acetic acid, a metabolite of 5-HT, 4-6 hours after the start of cisplatin [48]. This pattern of failure was not seen with ondansetron, and might indicate that the inital dose is sufficient and most relevant (Table 2). In a first study to investigate this hypothesis the loading dose of

Table 2. Efficacy of different doses/schedules of ondansetron in comparative studies

Dose (mg)	Schedule	No. evaluable pts.	Complete control (%)	Reference
8	bolus	173	52	Seynaeve et al. [50]
32	bolus	180	54	
8 + 24	bolus + CI	182	52	
32	bolus	154	58	Marty & D'Allens [49]
8 + 24	bolus + CI	151	57	
8	bolus	165	59	Ruff et al. [51]
32	bolus	162	51	
8	bolus	107	54	Beck et al. [52]
32	bolus	93	68	
0.15 mg/kg x 3	bolus	101	62	

8 mg followed by 24 mg given over 24 hours by continuous infusion was compared with 32 mg given as a short infusion [49]. No difference was observed in complete control of emesis: 57% (continuous infusion) versus 58% (single dose). Similar figures were found for nausea. In a second randomised, double-blind, parallel-group study (535 patients) no difference was found between 8 mg, 32 mg or continuous infusion (8 mg + 24 mg) [50]. Complete and major control was observed in 74% (continuous infusion), 78% (32 mg bolus) and 74% (8 mg bolus). The prognostic factors (cisplatin dose and gender) were well balanced over the 3 treatment groups. Analysis of these factors within this study showed that complete control of emesis was achieved in a significantly greater proportion of patients (65%) when cisplatin was given at a dose of <70 mg/m^2 in comparison to patients treated at a dose of ≥70 mg/m^2 (48%, $p < 0.001$). When only patients treated at a cisplatin dose of ≥100 mg/m^2 were analysed the percentage of complete responders was similar, namely 41-47%; however, the power to detect a difference was lower in view of the numbers involved. As might be expected, males did significantly better than females (67% versus 43%, $p < 0.001$). In a second European multicentre, double-blind, randomised, parallel-group study 2 doses of ondansetron were compared with 3 mg granisetron [51]. One hundred and sixty-five patients received 8 mg and 162 patients received 32 mg of ondansetron. Complete control was achieved in 59% of the patients treated with 8 mg and in 51% of the patients treated with 32 mg. Again no interaction between treatment and known prognostic factors was found in this study between the two dose levels. In the USA a similar study was performed comparing 32 mg with 8 mg and 0.15 mg/kg x 3 [52]. In this study a total of 699 patients were enrolled, receiving either high (≥ 100 mg/m^2) or intermediate (50-70 mg/m^2) doses of cisplatin. The 32 mg ondansetron dose was significantly better with regard to the total number of emetic episodes at the two cisplatin dose levels than the 8 mg and the 0.15 mg/kg x 3. With the presented data it is difficult to understand why there is a difference in outcome. The patients treated at a high cisplatin dose level were more numerous in the American study (more than 100 in each arm) than in the 3 European studies (less than 30 in all arms except one) and the European studies might have missed a difference in this subgroup due to a lack of power. However, this does not explain the difference at the intermediate dose level where the studies mentioned above are fully comparable with respect to patient characteristics.

The next question was whether the addition of corticosteroids would enhance the antiemetic efficacy of this new class of antiemetics. In a double-blind, multicentre, randomised cross-over study ondansetron (0.15 mg/kg x 3) was compared with the same schedule plus the addition of 20 mg dexamethasone. Eighty-nine patients completed both cycles, resulting in complete prevention of emesis in 64% of the ondansetron-alone group versus 91% of the combination group ($p = 0.0005$) [53]. Similar figures were found for nausea (89% versus

Table 3. The value of adding dexamethasone to ondansetron

Treatment	No. evaluable pts.	Complete control (%)	Reference
Ondansetron (0.15 mg/kg x 3)	48	64	Roila et al. [53]
Ondansetron + dexamethasone (20 mg)	54	92	
Ondansetron	27	30	Smith et al. [54]
Ondansetron + dexamethasone	27	78	
Ondansetron	71	40	Smyth et al. [55]
Ondansetron + dexamethasone	71	49	

66%, $p < 0.0025$). Complete protection from both nausea and vomiting was seen in 81% versus 56% of the patients ($p < 0.0008$). This observation was confirmed in 2 other studies (Table 3) [54,55].

The third-generation comparative studies include a comparison between the former best regimen with MCP and the current "best" regimen with ondansetron. The first study published showed a significantly better complete control of emesis for the ondansetron (0.15 mg/kg x 3) plus dexamethasone (20 mg) arm (78.7% versus 59.6%, $p < 0.002$) [56]. However, for nausea no significant difference was found (77.2% versus 65%, $p > 0.05$). Total prevention of nausea and vomiting was seen in 69% of the patients treated with the ondansetron combination versus 50% with the MCP combination. Of interest was the observation that patients receiving ondansetron on day 1 experienced significantly less vomiting on days 2 and 3 although the antiemetic regimen for both arms on these days was the same (oral MCP 20 mg x 4 and dexamethasone 8 mg i.m. twice daily on days 2, 3 and 4). It is also of interest to realise that the same regimen applied by the same group of investigators in a large group of patients resulted in a different percentage of patients who were completely protected from vomiting [53,56].

Almost all studies mentioned above are related to chemotherapy-naive patients and to the protection observed during the first 24 hours. Limited information is available on the maintenance of efficacy in subsequent courses. Most medical oncologists will support the "experience" that efficacy diminishes during subsequent courses. In a prospective double-blind, multicentre study the efficacy over 3 consecutive cycles was evaluated [56]. The results indicate a maintenance of efficacy for the ondansetron-treated patients with respect to the level of complete protection from emesis; this phenomenon was not observed in the MCP-treated group, were a decline from 59.6% to 47.5% occurred. For nausea there was a drop in efficacy in both treatment groups and in none of the 3 courses a significant difference was observed. A multifactorial logistic analysis of the prognostic factors indicated treatment, sex, dose of cisplatin and to a lesser extent age as clinically relevant factors in chemotherapy-naive patients. Protection during subsequent courses was clearly related to the achievement of complete protection during the first cycle. This emphasises once more the necessity to give the best treatment from the very beginning.

Other prospective studies comparing maintenance and efficacy over subsequent courses with combination antiemetic therapy including benzodiazepines, dexamethasone and MCP versus ondansetron and dexamethasone, are conducted but not yet published in peer-reviewed journals. More data will shortly be available to deepen our insights on this topic.

Ondansetron, Efficacy in Multiple-Day Cisplatin Regimens

The safety and efficacy of ondansetron in multiple-day courses was first shown in non-randomised studies [57,58]. In general the best responses were seen on day 1. The 5-HT$_3$ antagonists are relevant for these mainly young patients most often treated for germ-cell tumours, who are especially susceptible to the induction of extrapyramidal side-effects by MCP and are treated with curative intent. In a randomised, double-blind trial patients received MCP 1 mg/kg 3 times daily q 4 hours or ondansetron 3 times daily 0.15 mg/kg q 4 hours. The failure rate, defined as more than 5 emetic episodes during each 24-hour period, was significantly less in the ondansetron-treated group (9% versus 50%, $p = 0.002$) [59]. The difference in complete response rate on day 1 was also statistically significant in favour of ondansetron (78% versus 14%, $p < 0.001$). The differences on days 2 to 5 were not statistically significant, but the number of patients was low. As seen in the earlier non-randomised studies the efficacy of ondansetron decreased from 78% on day 1 to 57% on day 5; patients treated with MCP showed an inverse pattern with the highest reported protection on day 5 (50%). The observed level of protection of MCP is, however, surprisingly low and not in agreement with other observations. As might be expected, the incidence of extrapyramidal side-effects was high in the MCP-treated patients (59%). Also in the multiple-day regimens the addition of corticosteroids was shown to be useful [60]. In a randomised, open-label study 44 patients were treated with either ondansetron (0.15 mg/kg x 3 for 4 or 5 days) or ondansetron plus 2 days dexamethasone (8 mg at -30 min followed by 4 mg x 2 q 4 hours on days 1 and 2) and oral chlorpromazine (50 mg q 4 hours x 4 for 4 or 5 days). In the combination arm 86% of the patients experienced less than 3 emetic episodes throughout the study period compared with 46% in the ondansetron-alone arm ($p = 0.009$). The complete control rate was not different but this is probably due to the limited number of patients and the related insufficient power to detect a significant difference. The role of chlorpromazine in this schedule is not clear.

In a randomised, double-blind parallel-group study ondansetron (32 mg bolus) and dexamethasone (20 mg i.v.) was compared with MCP (2 or 1 mg/kg at -30 minutes +90 minutes) and dexamethasone in patients receiving multiple-day cisplatin therapy [61]. In this study no attempts were made to prevent extrapyramidal side-effects with diphenhydramine or piperidene. The dose of MCP was reduced from 2 to 1 mg/kg because 4 of the first 8 patients treated experienced extrapyramidal side-effects. The regimen of MCP given in this study is not optimal in view of the data available at that time. Seventy-one percent of the patients in the ondansetron plus dexamethasone arm experienced 2 or fewer emetic episodes over the entire 5-day period compared with 26% in the MCP group ($p < 0.001$).

Granisetron, Efficacy in Single-Day Cisplatin Regimens

Granisetron was shown to be safe in a wide dose range of 40 to 300 μg/kg [62]. In a dose ranging study from 2 to 160 μg/kg the dose of 2 μg/kg was clearly less effective than 10, 40 and 160 μg/kg, suggesting a broad range of efficacy with loss of protection below 10 μg/kg [63]. From the very beginning a single-dose regimen was explored with initially a provision for an additional two doses over the next 24 hours provided that the patients suffered from severe nausea and vomiting. The definitions used in the granisetron studies are slightly different from those used in the other antiemetic studies. Complete control was defined as no nausea or vomiting or only mild nausea in the 24 hours after chemotherapy, major control was defined as a single vomiting episode in the first 24 hours or no vomiting but moderate to severe nausea, and the registration of more than 4 vomiting episodes in the first 24 hours was considered as failure. In a double-blind, randomised dose-finding study in chemotherapy-naive patients treated with cisplatin ($\geq$50 mg/m^2) 2 levels of granisetron (40 and 160 μg/kg) were compared with the allowance of the earlier mentioned two additional doses of 40 μg/kg [64]. A total of 335 patients were randomised and no difference could be found (complete responders 57% and 59%, respectively). The single dose of 40 μg/kg was used for subsequent comparative trials. In a single-blind randomised study 40 μg/kg granisetron given as a 5-minute infusion completed 5 minutes before the start of cisplatin was compared with high-dose MCP given as a loading dose of 3 mg/kg followed by a maintenance of 4 mg/kg given over 8 hours plus dexamethasone 12 mg [65]. A total of 281 patients were randomised, all but 4 patients were chemotherapy naive (cisplatin ≥50 mg/m2). In 70% of the granisetron-treated patients complete control was obtained; this was similar for the MCP + dexamethasone-treated group with 68%. For the subgroup of patients receiving a cisplatin dose of over 100 mg/m2 these results were similar. The dose of 40 μg/kg has been "translated" to 3 mg and is considered the recommended dose. In view of the available data, 1 mg can probably be considered as equally effective.

Granisetron, Efficacy in Multiple-Day Cisplatin Regimens

In one large single-blind randomised study [66] granisetron (40 μg/kg) was compared with alizapride (4 mg/kg prior to the start of cisplatin followed by 4 mg/kg at 4 and 8 hours post-treatment) plus dexamethasone (8 mg). In the granisetron-treated group a complete control over 5 days was seen in 49.3% (n=72) of the patients versus 35.4% (n=63) for the alizapride plus dexamethasone group. These differences were not significant, as might be expected in view of the number of patients involved. Efficacy (complete control) on day 1 in the granisetron-treated patients was significantly better (90.3% versus 65.9%, $p < 0.001$).

Tropisetron, Efficacy in Single-Day Cisplatin Regimens

In a dose-ranging study (12-48 mg/m2) no dose-limiting toxicity was observed [67]. In a double-blind randomised study with a total of 100 patients treated with cisplatin, 4 different single doses of tropisetron were explored: 5 mg, 10 mg, 20 mg and 40 mg. Tropisetron was given as an intravenous infusion over 15 minutes prior to cisplatin administration. Overall, 54% total protection from vomiting and nausea was reported. No dose-response relation was found and between the numbers studied at the various dose levels no differences could be found [68]. In the group of patients treated with 100 mg/m2 cisplatin the level of total protection was 40%. In a single-centre double-blind study tropisetron was compared with MCP (20 mg/m2 i.v. followed by MCP orally 10 mg/m2 3 times daily) plus dexamethasone (10 mg/m2 i.v.) [69]. Tropisetron treatment was started with a 5 mg tablet the evening before and 5 mg i.v. just prior to the start of the cisplatin infusion and continued the next morning with an additional tablet of 5 mg. In the tropisetron-treated group 76% of the patients (n=57) experienced total protection from vomiting in contrast to 39% in the MCP plus dexamethasone group (n=57). The dose of MCP used in this study is insufficient in view of the reported experience in the literature. In a multicentre randomised study involving cisplatin-treated patients tropisetron 5 mg i.v. followed by 5 mg orally once a day on days 2 to 4 was compared with dexamethasone 8 mg i.v., then 4 mg i.v. q 6 hours x 4 and MCP 3 mg/kg i.v. followed by 4 mg/kg continuous infusion over 8 hours then 20 mg orally, 3 times a day, on days 2-4 [70]. In this study MCP plus dexamethasone was superior to tropisetron (53% versus 34% no vomiting, $p = 0.04$).

Comparative Studies

Several studies have addressed the question whether the earlier mentioned differences in the pharmacological and pre-clinical features between the three compounds discussed result in a clinically relevant difference [51,71-73].

In a double-blind crossover study granisetron and ondansetron were compared in 5-day fractionated chemotherapy (84% cisplatin and 16% ifosfamide) [71]. Patients received either a 3-times intravenous dose of 8 mg ondansetron or a once-daily dose of 3 mg granisetron. A total of 309 out of 359 patients completed the 2-way crossover study. The complete response rate (mild nausea included) was similar for both drugs (90%), however, 34% of the patients preferred granisetron, 25.6% preferred ondansetron ($p<0.05$) and 39.2% expressed no preference. Toxicity was equivalent and an objective reason for the difference in preference is lacking so far. A second study, which has been mentioned before [51], compared two dose levels of ondansetron (8 and 32 mg) with 3 mg granisetron. In this study 496 patients were randomised and no difference in complete control of emesis was found between the 3 arms tested (59%, 51% and 56%, respectively). A similar pattern was seen when complete and major control were analysed. Nausea (none or mild) was recorded in 69% of the ondansetron-treated patients and 73% in the granisetron-treated group. There were no significant differences between the treatment groups when global satisfaction scores were compared. No interaction was found between treatments and prognostic factors on complete or major control. No differences were recorded with respect to drug-related adverse events.

In 2 open, randomised, single-institution studies [72] 2 doses of ondansetron given as a single intravenous infusion (24 mg, n = 182 and 16 mg, n = 164) were compared with 3 mg granisetron. No difference in complete response was reported (52% for O and 49% for G in study 1 and 69% for O and 67% for G in study 2). In a recently presented large randomised study [73] 8 mg ondansetron was compared with 3 mg granisetron; both compounds were combined with 20 mg dexamethasone. A total of 973 patients were entered with 966 patients evaluable. Complete protection from acute vomiting and nausea was obtained in 79.3% and 72% of the ondansetron-treated patients versus 79.9% and 71.8% of the granisetron-treated patients. This study would have been able to detect a 10% difference with a power of 80%. To detect smaller if at all relevant differences thousands of patients should be enrolled in double-blind, randomised trials. The data of non-randomised studies are insufficient to draw conclusions with respect to difference or equivalence between the available compounds. Based on the available data there is no relevant difference in efficacy for acute cisplatin-induced emesis between the two most studied agents and the choice of either of the two will probably be based on subjective and secondary factors such as patient preference, costs and availability.

Side-Effects of 5-HT_3 Antagonists

For all three compounds discussed the toxicity profile is excellent. The most important side-effects are headache and constipation but these are rarely of any clinical relevance and can be controlled with simple medication if at all indicated.

With ondansetron headache is the most frequently reported adverse effect, having an incidence of up to 43% [74]. Constipation has been observed in approximately 10% of the patients and is related to its effect on gut motility; diarrhoea has been seen in up to 22% of the patients. The incidence of liver function abnormalities varies and might be related to the cisplatin medication and not to ondansetron. In the randomised studies the incidence of liver function abnormalities in the ondansetron and control arms were similar [40-41]. The liver function abnormalities observed so far are asymptomatic and transient. A surprising observation has been the occurrence of extrapyramidal reactions after the administration of ondansetron [75,76]. The number of patients treated with the other representatives of this class of antiemetics is smaller and this side-effect has not been reported with granisetron or tropisetron. It is too early to state that this side-effect can be mediated via the 5-HT_3 receptor. In ondansetron it has been shown that there is some binding with other receptors [36], which could be involved in the induction of this side-effect. The incidence is very low but should be recognised and treated accordingly. With respect to tolerability no clear dose relationship has been observed [49,52].

The tolerability profile of granisetron is very similar to that of ondansetron, with headache in about 10-15% of patients, constipation (0-4%) and rarely diarrhoea [76]. Transient, clinically insignificant changes in blood pressure have been observed.

For tropisetron the same pattern of side-effects has been observed [78]. In addition, 4 patients receiving doses of 25 and 50 mg developed skin reactions such as pruritis, rash, exanthema and urticaria, and in 2 patients with a carcinoid syndrome arthralgia was seen. One of these patients also developed a transient lymphadenopathy.

Future Perspectives

When we consider the data discussed above it is obvious that an important step forward has been made. On the other hand, complete protection during the first 24 hours for all patients is still an illusion and this is especially the case for young women receiving highly emetogenic chemotherapy. Furthermore, protection during subsequent courses, although good in a few studies during the first 3 courses, is a relevant

Table 4. Dose and schedule of granisetron, ondansetron and tropisetron

Drug	Route	Infusion time	Time point	Dose	Schedule
Granisetron	i.v.	5 min	t - 10 min	3 mg (1 mg)	1 x
Ondansetron	i.v	15 min	t - 30 min	8 mg (32 mg)	1 x
Tropisetron	i.v.	5 min	t - 5 min	5 mg 5 mg tablet day 2	1 x

problem. Oral formulations of the above-mentioned compounds are available and currently under investigation; in view of the supposed site of action their efficacy may be equivalent to the intravenous formulations. Steps to improve on the present achievements could be blockade of other receptors involved in the emetic reflex such as the dopamine D_2 receptor. In a recent crossover study the addition of metopimazine, a selective dopamine D_2 antagonist, resulted in a significantly reduced incidence of both acute and delayed nausea and vomiting [79]. Ondansetron was given orally 8 mg twice a day and metopimazine was given in 30 mg tablets 4 times a day. All medication was given for 3 days. Thirty previously treated patients who vomited at least once during the previous chemotherapy, were studied and the chemotherapy was moderately emetogenic. It was postulated that this combination might be of special relevance for the delayed phase where serotonin antagonists seem less effective. This study gives no definite proof of the value of this combination but this observation should be further explored.

Conclusions

In view of the data presented, 5-HT_3 antagonists should be regarded as first-line treatment for the prevention of cisplatin-induced emesis. The optimal doses and schedules are presented in Table 4. Based on 2 large European studies the recommended dose for ondansetron is a single i.v. dose of 8 mg. According to the American data 32 mg should be considered. The treatment of choice for granisetron is 3 mg and for tropisetron 5 mg. In case of high-dose cisplatin, at least above 50 mg/m^2, corticosteroids should be added. The optimal dose is not known, efficacy has been observed between 8 and 50 mg for dexamethasone and 250 and 1000 mg for methylprednisolone. When low doses of cisplatin are used the above-mentioned dosages can be used without the addition of corticosteroids.

REFERENCES

1 Seynaeve C, de Mulder PHM, Verweij J, Gralla RJ: Controlling cancer chemotherapy-induced emesis. An update. Pharm Weekbl [Sci] 1991 (13):189-197

2 Allen SG, Smith SF: Small intestinal toxicity of cisplatin - comparison of effects of platinum analogues and dexamethasone. Br J Cancer 1986 (53):355-360

3 Akwari OE: The gastrointestinal tract in chemotherapy induced emesis. Drugs 1983 (25):18-34

4 Schwörer H, Racke K, Kilbinger H: Cisplatin increases the release of 5-hydroxytryptamine from the isolated vascularly perfused small intestine of the guinea pig: Involvement of 5HT3 receptors. Naunyn-Schmiedeberg's Arch Pharmacol 1991 (344):143-149

5 Miner WD, Sanger G: Inhibition of cisplatin induced vomiting by selective 5-hydroxytryptamine M-receptor antoganism. Br J Parmacol 1986 (88):497-499

6 Gralla RJ, Itri LM, Pisko SE et al: Antiemetic efficacy of high-dose metoclopramide: randomised trials with placebo and prochlorperazine in patients with chemotherapy induced nausea and vomiting. N Engl J Med 1981 (305):905-909

7 Craig JB, Powell BL: Review: The management of nausea and vomiting in clinical oncology. Am J Med Sci 1987 (293): 34-44

8 Grunberg SM, Gala KV, Lampenfield M et al: Comparison of the antiemitic efficacy of high-dose intravenous metoclopramide and high-dose intravenous haloperidol in randomized double-blind crossover study. J Clin Oncol 1984 (2):782-787

9 Saller R, Hellenbrecht D: High doses of metoclopramide or droperidol in the prevention of cisplatin induced emesis. Eur J Cancer Clin Oncol 1986 (22):1199-1203

10 Basurto C, Roila F, Del Favero A: A prospective randomised double blind crossover study comparing the antiemetic effect of alizapride and metoclopramide in patients receiving cisplatin chemotherapy. Cancer Invest (1988):475-479

11 Saller R, Hellenbrecht D: Comparision of the antiemetic efficacy of 2 high-dose benzamides, metoclopramide and alizapride, against cisplatin induced emesis. Cancer Treatm Rep 1985 (69):1301-1302

12 Frustaci S, Grattoni E, Tumolo S et al: Randomised crossover antiemetic study in cisplatin treated patients. Cancer Chemother Pharmacol 1986 (17): 75-79

13 Meyer BR, Levin M, Draper DE et al: Optimising metoclopramide control of cisplatin induced emesis. Ann Intern Med 1984 (100):393-395

14 Kerr PJ, Graham J, McGovern E et al: The relationship between steady state metoclopramide levels and control of emesis during treatment with cisplatinum. Br J Clin Pharm 11985 (20):426-427

15 Mc Dermed JE, Cohen JL, Joseph C, Strum SB: Clinical pharmacokinetics of high-dose metoclopramide in cancer patients receiving cisplatin therapy. J Clin Oncol 1985 (3):1400-1408

16 Grundberg SM, Mc Dermed JE, Berstein L, Cohen JL: Examination of the correlation of serum MCP levels with antiemetic efficacy in patients receiving cisplatin. Cancer Chemoth Pharmac 1987 (20):332-336

17 Kris MG, Gralla RJ, Clark RA et al: Antiemetic control and prevention of side effects of anticancer therapy with lorazepam when used in combination with metoclopramide and dexamethasone. Cancer 1987 (60):2816-2822

18 Anthony L, Krozeby M, Woodward et al: Antiemetic effecacy of oral versus intravenous MCP in patients receiving cisplatin. J Clin Oncol 1985 (4):98-103

19 Warrington PS, Allan SG, Cornbleet MA, MacPherson JS, Smyth JF, Leonard RCF: Optimising antiemesis in cancer chemotherapy: efficacy of continuous versus intermittent infusion of high dose metoclopramide in emesis induced by cisplatin. Br Med J 1986 (293):1334-1337

20 Parashos PJ, Dugan WM, Fry MW: Continuous infusion metoclopramide: clinical trials, pharmacokinetic considerations and cost effectiviness. In: Engstrom PF, Mortenson LE, Anderson PN (eds). Progress in Clinical and Biological Research. A. Liss, New York 1987 p 303

21 Agostinucci, WA, Gannon RH, Schauer PK, Walters JK: Continuous infusion of metoclopramide for prevention of chemotherapy induced emesis. Clin Pharmacology 1986 (5): 150-153

22 Navari RM: Comparision of intermittent versus continuous infusion metoclopramide in control of acute nausea induced by cisplatin chemotherapy. J Clin Oncol 1989 (7): 943-946

23 Tyson LB, Gralla RJ, Kris MG, Young CW, Clark RA: Dose-ranging antiemetic trial of high-dose oral MCP. Am J Clin Oncol (1989):239-243

24 Anthony L, Krozeby M, Woodward et al: Antiemetic efficacy of oral versus intravenous MCP in patients receiving cisplatin. J Clin Oncol 1985 (4):98-103

25 Allan SG, Cornbleet MA, Warrington PS et al: Dexamethasone and high dose metoclopramide: Efficacy in controlling cisplatin-induced nausea and vomiting. Br Med J 1984 (289):878-879

26 Rosell R, Abad-Esteve A, Ribas-Mundo M et al: Evaluation of a combination antiemetic regimen including i.v. high-dose metoclopramide, dexamethasone, and diphenhydramine in cisplatin-based chemotherapy regimens. Cancer Treat Rep 1985 (69):909-910

27 Roila F, Tonato M, Basurto C et al: Antiemetic activity of high dose of metoclopramide combined with methylprednisolone versus metoclopramide alone in cisplatin-treated cancer patients. J Clin Oncol 1987 (5):141-149

28 Cognetti F, Carlini P, Pinnaro P et al: Maintenance of antiemetic effect of a MCP/Dex combination during subsequent cisplatin courses. Oncology 1986 (43): 292-294

29 Aapro MS: Present role of corticosteroids as antiemetics. In: Senn H-J and Glaus A (eds) Recent Results in Cancer Research. Springer-Verlag, Berlin Heidelberg 1991 pp 91-100

30 Kearsley JH, Williams AM, Fiumara AM: Antiemetic superiority of lorazepam over oxazepam and methylprednisolone as premedicants for patients receiving cisplatin-containing chemotherapy. Cancer 1989 (64):1595-1599

31 Bishop JF, Olver IN, Wolf MM et al: Lorazepam: a randomised, double-blind, crossover study of a new antiemetic in patients receiving cytotoxic chemotherapy and prochlorperazine. J Clin Oncol 1984 (2): 691-695
32 Gordon CJ, Pasdur R, Zicarelli A, Cummings G, Al-Sarraf M: Metoclopramide versus metoclopramide and lorazepam. Cancer 1989 (63):578-582
33 Kriss MG, Gralla RJ, Tyson LB et al: Improved control of cisplatin induced emesis with high-dose metoclopramide and with combinations of metoclopramide, dexamethasone and diphenhydramine. Cancer 1985 (55):527-534
34 Seynaeve C, Verweij J, de Mulder PHM: 5 HT3 receptor antagonists. A new approach in emesis. A review of ondansetron, granisetron and tropisetron. Anti Cancer Drugs 1991 (19):203-208
35 Tyers MB, Freeman AJ: Mechanism of the anti-emetic activity of 5-HT3 receptor antagonists. Oncology 1992 (49):263-268
36 Andrew PLR, Bhandari P, Davey PT, Bingham S, Marr HE, Blower PR: Are all 5-T3 receptor antagonists the same? Eur J Cancer 1992 (28A suppl 1): s2-s6
37 Aapro MS: '... Setron'?: Are 5-HT3 receptor antagonists different? Eur J Cancer 1993 (29a):1655
38 Perez EA: Review of the preclinical pharmacology and comparative efficacy of 5-hydroxytryptamine-3 receptor antagonists for chemotherapy-induced emesis. J Clin Oncol 1995 (13):1036-1043
39 De Haan LD, de Mulder PHM, Beex LVAM et al: The efficacy of GR38032F, an antagonist of 5-hydroxytryptamine-3 (5-HT3) in the prophylaxis of cisplatin (CDDP)-induced nausea and vomiting. Eur J Cancer Clin Oncol 1988 (24):1383-1384
40 Marty M, Pouillart P, Scholl S, Droz JP, Azab M, Brion N, Pujade-Lauraine E, Paule B, Paes D, Bons J: Comparision of the 5-hydroxytryptamine, (serotonin) antagonist ondansetron (GR 38032F) with high-dose metoclopramide in the control of cisplatin-induced emesis. N Engl J Med 1990 (322): 816-821
41 De Mulder PHM, Seynaeve C, Vermorken JB, van Liessum PA, Mols-Jevdevic S, Lane Allman E, Beranek P, Verweij J: Ondansetron compared with high-dose metoclopramide in prophylaxis of acute and delayed cisplatin-induced nausea and vomiting. Ann Intern Med 1990 (113):834-840
42 Kris MG, Gralla RJ, Clark RA, Tyson LB: Dose-ranging evaluation of the serotonin antagonist GR38032F when used as an antiemetic in patients recieving anticancer therapy. J Clin Oncol 1988 (6):659-662
43 Grundberg SM, Stevenson LL, Russell CA, McDermed JE: Dose ranging phase I study of the serotonin antagonist GR38032F for prevention of cisplatin-induced nausea and vomiting. J Clin Oncol 1989 (7):1137-1141
44 Kris MG, Gralla RJ, Clark RA, Tyson LB: Phase II trials of the serotonin antagonist GR38032F for the control of vomiting caused by cisplatin. JNCI 1989 (81):42-46
45 Hesketh PJ, Murphy WK, Lester EP et al: GR38032F: a novel compound effective in the prevention of acute cisplatin-induced emesis. J Clin Oncol 1989 (7):700-705
46 Khojasteh A, Sartiano G, Tapazoglou E et al: Ondansetron for the prevention of emesis induced by high-dose cisplatin. Cancer 1990 (66):1101-1105
47 Hainsworth J, Harvey W, Pendergrass K et al: A single-blind comparison of intravenous ondansetron, a selective serotonin antagonist, with intravenous metoclopramide in the prevention of nausea and vomiting associated with high-dose cisplatin chemotherapy. J Clin Oncol 1991 (9):721-728
48 Cubeddu LX, Hoffmann IS, Fuenmayor NT, Finn AL: Efficacy of ondansetron and the role of serotonin in cisplatin-induced nausea and vomiting. N Engl J Med 1990 (322):810-816
49 Marty M, D'Allens H: Etude randomisée en double-insu comparant l'efficacité de l'ondansetron selon deux modes d'administration: injection unique et perfusion continue. Cahiers Cancer 1990 (2): 541-546
50 Seynaeve C, Schuller J, Buser K et al: Comparision of the anti-emetic efficacy of different doses of ondansetron, given as either a continuous infusion or a single intravenous dose, in acute cisplatin-induced emesis. A multicentre, double-blind, randomised, parallel group study. Br J Cancer 1992 (66):192-197
51 Ruff P, Paska W, Goedhals L et al: Ondansetron compared with granisetron in the prophylaxis of cisplatin-induced acute emesis: a multicentre double-blind, randomised, parallel-group study. Oncology 1994 (51):113-118
52 Beck Th M, Hesketh PJ, Madajewicz S et al: Stratified, randomized, double-blind comparision of intravenous ondansetron administered as a multiple-dose regimen versus two single-dose regimens in the prevention of cisplatin-induced nausea and vomiting. J Clin Oncol 1992 (10):1969-1975
53 Roila F, Tonato M, Cognetti F et al: Prevention of cisplatin-induced emesis: a double-blind multicenter randomized crossover study comparing ondansetron and ondansetron plus dexamethasone. J Clin Oncol 1991 (9):675-678
54 Smith DB, Newlands ES, Rustin GJS et al: Comparison of ondansetron and ondansetron plus dexamethasone as antiemetic prophylaxis during cisplatin-containing chemotherapy. Lancet 1991 (338):487-490
55 Smyth JF, Coleman RE, Nicolson M et al: Does dexamethasone enhance control of acute cisplatin induced emesis by ondansetron? Br Med J 1991 (303):1423-1426
56 Italian Group for Antiemetic Research: Difference in persistence of efficacy of two antiemetic regimens on acute emesis during cisplatin chemotherapy. J Clin Oncol 1993 (11):2396-2404
57 Kris MG, Gralla RJ, Clark RA et al: Phase II trials of the serotonin antagonist GR38032F for the control of vomiting caused by cisplatin. JNCI 1989 (81):42-46
58 Hainsworth JD: The use of ondansetron in patients receiving multiple-day cisplatin regimens. Sem Oncol 1992 (19 suppl 10):48-52
59 Sledge GW, Einhorn LH, Nagy C et al: Phase III double-blind comparison of intravenous ondanse-

tron and metoclopramide as antiemetic therapy for patients receiving multiple-day cisplatin-based chemotherapy. Cancer 1992 (70):2524-2528
60 Fox SM, Einhorn LH, Cox E, Powell N, Abdy A: Ondansetron versus ondansetron, dexamethasone, and chlorpromazine in the prevention of nausea and vomiting associated with multiple-day cisplatin chemotherapy. J Clin Oncol 1993 (11):2391-2395
61 Räth U, Upadhyaya BK, Arechavala E et al: Role of ondansetron plus dexamethasone in fractionated chemotherapy. Oncology 1993 (50):168-172
62 Upward JW, Arnold BDC, Link C et al: The clinical pharmacology of granisetron (BRL43694A), a novel specific 5-HT3 antagonist. Eur J Cancer 1990 (26 suppl 1):S12-S15
63 Kamanabrou D, on behalf of the Granisetron Study Group: Intravenous granisetron - establishing the optimal dose. Eur J Cancer 1992 (28A suppl 1):S6-11
64 Soukop M, on behalf of the Granisetron Study Group: A comparison of two dose levels of granisetron in patients recieving high-dose cisplatin. Eur J Cancer 1990 (29 suppl 1):S15-S19
65 Chevallier B, on behalf of the Granisetron Study Group: The control of acute cisplatin-induced emesis - a comparative study of granisetron and a combination regimen of high-dose metoclopramide and dexamethasone. Br J Cancer 1993 (68):176-180
66 Bremer K, on behalf of the Granisetron Study Group: A single-blind study of the efficacy and safety of intravenous granisetron compared with alizapride plus dexamethasone in the prophylaxis and control of emesis in patients receiving 5-day cytostatic therapy. Eur J Cancer 1992 (28A no 6/7):1018-1022
67 Tyson LR, Gralla RJ, Kris MG, Clark RA: Phase I antiemetic study of the serotonin antagonist ICS 205-930. Proc Am Soc Clin Oncol 1989 (8):331
68 Stamatakis L, Michel J, Van Belle S et al: ICS 205-930: A dose finding study in the prevention of cisplatin induced nausea and vomiting. Proc Am Soc Clin Oncol 1989 (8):327
69 Krzakowski M, Madaj G, Pawinsky A et al: A comparative study of the use of Novaban, a 5-HT antagonist, versus a standard anti-emetic regimen of dexamethasone and metoclopramide in the treatment of chemotherapy-induced emesis. Ann Oncol 1992 (3):155-161
70 Kris MG, Tyson LB: Tropisetron (ICS 205-930): A selective 5-hydroxtryptamine antagonist. Eur J Cancer 1993 (29A suppl 1):30-32
71 Noble A, Bremer K, Dilly SG et al: A double blind, crossover comparison of granisetron and ondansetron in 5-day fractionated chemotherapy: Assessment of efficacy, safety, and patient preference. Eur J Cancer 1994 (30A):1083-1088
72 Gebbia V, Cannata G, Testa A et al: Ondansetron versus granisetron in the prevention of chemotherapy-induced nausea and vomiting. Results of a prospective randomized trial. Cancer 1994 (74):1945-1952
73 Roila F, De Angelis V, Cognetti F et al: Ondansetron versus granisetron, both combined with dexamethasone in the prevention of cisplatin-induced emesis. Proc Am Soc Clin Oncol 1995 (14):523
74 Chaffee BJ, Tankanow RM: Drug Review. Ondansetron - the first of a new class of antiemetic agents. Clin Pharm 1991 (10):430-446
75 Halperin JR, Murphy B: Extrapyramidal reaction on ondansetron. Cancer 1992 (69):1275
76 Jacobsen MBJ: Ondansetron in carcinoid syndrome. Lancet 1992 (340):185
77 Plosker GL, Goa KL: Granisetron. A review of its pharmacological properties and therapeutic use as an antiemetic. Drugs 1991 (42):805-824
78 de Bruijn KM: Tropisetron. A review of the clinical experience. Drugs 1992 (43):11-22
79 Herrstedt J, Sigsgaard T, Boesgaard M et al: Ondansetron plus metopimazine compared with ondansetron alone in patients receiving moderately emetogenic chemotherapy. N Engl J Med 1993 (328):1076-1081

Prevention of Acute Emesis from Other Emetogenic Drugs

Miguel Martin and Eduardo Díaz-Rubio

Servicio de Oncología Médica, Hospital Universitario San Carlos, 28040 Madrid, Spain

Although cisplatin is the most emetogenic cytotoxic agent, many other antineoplastic drugs are also able to induce moderate to severe emesis. Table 1 shows a ranking of the emetic potential of several antitumour agents different from cisplatin. It is important to point out that the final intensity of emesis is not only related to the intrinsic emetic capacity of the antitumour drug, but to other prognostic factors such as gender of the patient, previous chemotherapy-induced emesis, age, route, dose, schedule and setting of administration of the agent, combination with other emetic drugs, etc. [1,2].

In a seminal work by Kris et al. [3], acute emesis was defined as emesis occurring during the first 24 hours after cisplatin, and delayed emesis as nausea and vomiting beginning 24 hours or more after chemotherapy administration. The distinction of delayed emesis as a separate entity was initially applied to cisplatin-induced emesis, and has found substantial support by the fact that it is not easily controlled by means of antiserotoninergic agents [4], thus suggesting a pathogenic mechanism different from that of the acute phase. The concept of delayed emesis has been extended in many recent studies to emesis induced by other antineoplastic agents, including carboplatin and cyclophosphamide. A number of studies have shown that these two drugs, as well as their combinations, induce a special pattern of emesis which is characterised by a late onset of vomiting (6-12 hours after chemotherapy) followed by an uninterrupted period of nausea and vomiting lasting, in nearly one-third of patients, for 2 or more days [5-7]. The delayed phase of cyclophosphamide or carboplatin-induced vomiting usually responds to antiserotoninergic antiemetics, and so does the acute phase [8-10]. For this reason, the consideration of delayed emesis as a distinct entity is controversial in the case of emesis induced by non-cisplatin containing combinations, and could create difficulties in the interpretation of the results of antiemetic trials [7].

Therefore, our review will focus on the overall control of emesis provoked by non-cisplatin containing combinations (i.e., control over days 1 through 5) rather than the control of the acute phase of emesis.

The denomination "non-cisplatin containing chemotherapy" or "moderately emetogenic chemotherapy" includes a potpourri of different drugs and combinations with diverse emetogenic capacity and emetic patterns. Many recent trials have tested the activity of the new antiemetic agents in heterogeneous popula-

Table 1. Emetogenic potential of antitumour drugs other than cisplatin (i.v. route)

Drug	Emetogenic potential
Dacarbazine	+
Dactinomycin	▲
Mechloretamine	│
Streptozocin	│
Ifosfamide	│
Carboplatin	│
Cyclophosphamide	│
Nitrosoureas	│
Doxorubicin	│
Cytarabine	│
Daunorubicin	│
Epirubicin	│
Methotrexate	│
Mitomycin C	│
Mitoxantrone	│
5-Fluorouracil	│
Teniposide	│
Etoposide	│
Taxol	│
Bleomycin	│
Vinca alkaloids	–

tions of patients treated with different chemotherapy regimens, including combinations of DTIC, carboplatin, cyclophosphamide, doxorubicin, epirubicin and other moderately emetogenic cytotoxic agents [11-13]. These trials can provide a preliminary and general idea of the clinical activity of the new antiemetics. However, more refined studies addressing the issue of emetic control in a specific patient population (e.g. female patients treated with FAC chemotherapy) are needed in order to obtain clear guidelines for the management of emesis in specific groups of patients. Consequently, our review will pay special attention to studies addressing the control of emesis provoked by specific chemotherapy regimens.

Cyclophospamide

Cyclophosphamide is widely used in the treatment of solid tumours, usually in combination with other cytotoxic drugs such as anthracyclines, methotrexate, vincristine and 5-fluorouracil. The incidence of emesis after cyclophosphamide seems to be dose-dependent, ranging from 50-70% at conventional intravenous doses (500-600 mg/m^2) to nearly 100% with high-dose regimens (50-75 mg/kg) [5,14].

The pattern of emesis after both conventional [15] and high-dose [5] cyclophosphamide is very different from that of cisplatin. In patients treated with placebo or uneffective antiemetics, the onset of emesis occurs between 6 and 12 hours after cyclophosphamide administration. Vomiting subsides after 24 hours in approximately 75% of the patients, although nausea persists for 2 to 3 days in some patients.

A number of studies have addressed the control of emesis provoked by i.v. cyclophosphamide in miscellaneous populations of patients treated with this drug in association with other cytotoxics of diverse emetogenic capacity. Ondansetron has proven to be effective in the control of nausea and vomiting induced by combinations containing i.v. cyclophosphamide (500 mg/m^2 or more) and other cytotoxic agents. In a preliminary study on 55 patients receiving ondansetron (8 mg orally tds for 3 to 5 days), complete and major control of vomiting on day 1 was observed in 94.5% of patients and nausea was graded as absent or mild in 83.3% of cases on the same day. The complete and major control rate improved on subsequent study days from 96.1% on study day 2 to 100% on study day 5 [8].

In a randomised, double-blind, placebo-controlled study ondansetron (0.15 mg/kg i.v. 30 min prior to chemotherapy and 4 and 8 hours later) was clearly superior to placebo in the control of emesis induced by cyclophosphamide (500 to 600 mg/m^2 i.v.) in combination with other drugs (methotrexate, doxorubicin, 5-fluorouracil, vincristine and dacarbazine) [15]. During the 24-hour period after cyclophosphamide, 70% of the patients treated with ondansetron versus 0% of the patients given a placebo were completely free of vomiting. The control of emesis on days 2 to 5 with ondansetron was similar to day 1 (70% of complete responders).

Herrstedt et al. [16] reported the results of a randomised, double-blind, crossover study comparing ondansetron (8 mg per os before chemotherapy and then every 8 hours for 3 days) with ondansetron (same dose) plus the dopamine D_2 antagonist metopimazine (30 mg per os 4 times a day for 3 days) in breast cancer patients who had presented some degree of vomiting in previous courses of cyclophosphamide containing chemotherapy. The association was superior to ondansetron alone in the control of emesis on day 1 (63% versus 47% of complete responders), on days 2 through 5 (73% versus 50%) and on days 1 through 5 (53% versus 43%).

The antiemetic efficacy of a single i.v. dose of granisetron (40 µg/kg) has also been assessed in a randomised, single-blind, parallel-group study comparing this 5-HT_3 antagonist with the combination of chlorpromazine plus dexamethasone in patients receiving moderately emetogenic chemotherapy [17]. Overall, granisetron was superior to chlorpromazine plus dexamethasone in the control of emesis on day 1. In the subset of patients receiving cyclophosphamide containing combinations, a complete control of emesis on day 1 was observed in 61% of patients receiving granisetron versus 42% of patients receiving chlorpromazine plus dexamethasone. Emetic control on days 2-7 was not specifically reported for the cyclophosphamide-treated population.

The emetic capacity of cyclophosphamide containing chemotherapy regimens, however, is clearly influenced by the associated drugs. The combination of i.v. cyclophosphamide, doxorubicin and 5-fluorouracil (FAC) is more emetogenic than the CMF regimen, in which doxorubicin is substituted by methotrexate, a less emetogenic drug. Therefore, the analysis of studies addressing the control of emesis provoked by specific types of cyclophosphamide containing combinations (e.g. CMF or FAC), rather than by miscellaneous cyclophosphamide containing combinations, will provide more practical and precise guidelines for the management of emesis in such particular subsets of patients.

Classic (standard) CMF

This regimen is widely used for the adjuvant treatment of breast cancer and consists of oral cyclophosphamide (100 mg/m^2/day on days 1 through 14), i.v. 5-fluorouracil (600 mg/m^2 on days 1 and 8) and i.v. methotrexate (40 mg/m^2 on days 1 and 8). In a prospective evaluation of 55 patients after the fourth cycle of classical CMF, 62% reported mild or marked nausea and/or vomiting [18]. Therefore, some kind of antiemetic prophylaxis seems necessary for this moderately emetogenic regimen.

Buser et al. [19] compared oral ondansetron (8 mg every 8 hours on days 1 through 15) with placebo in 80 breast cancer patients receiving the classic CMF regimen. Sixty-three percent of patients treated with ondansetron and 29% of patients treated with placebo reported no vomiting or retching during the 15-day study period ($p<0.01$).

Levitt et al. [20] carried out a double-blind, parallel-group, multicentre trial involving 165 breast cancer patients due to receive classic CMF. In this trial the antiemetic efficacy of oral ondansetron (8 mg every 8 hours on days 1 through 7) was compared with that of a combination of a single dose of dexamethasone (10 mg i.v. prior to i.v. chemotherapy) and oral metoclopramide (10 mg every 8 hours on days 1 through 7). There were no statistically significant differences in terms of control of vomiting between the two arms. More than 66% of the patients did not vomit during the 7-day study period. The group given dexamethasone-metoclopramide experienced less nausea during the first 24 hours of the study, even though the differences between the 7-day averages of nausea scores were only of borderline significance ($p=0.08$).

Taking into account the cost of ondansetron given over prolonged periods of time (14-15 days), which largely exceeds the cost of CMF chemotherapy itself, the combination of i.v. dexamethasone and oral metoclopramide seems to be at the present time the best antiemetic choice for breast cancer patients receiving standard CMF. Further refinements in antiemetic prophylaxis are needed for these patients, since nearly one-third still experience some degree of vomiting with dexamethasone-metoclopramide.

Intravenous CMF

This regimen is a modification of the standard CMF protocol. Cyclophosphamide (600 mg/m^2), methotrexate (40 mg/m^2) and 5-fluorouracil (600 mg/m^2) are given by intravenous route on day 1 every 3 weeks. In placebo-treated patients, i.v. CMF induces some degree of emesis in 70-72% of patients [21,22]. The median latency time of nausea and vomiting is 9 hours (range 6-18 hours), and vomits can persist for 24-48 hours [21]. Perhaps because of this emetic pattern, a short course of high-dose i.v. metoclopramide (1 mg/kg before and 1 mg/kg 30 minutes after chemotherapy) was not superior to placebo in the control of i.v. CMF-induced emesis [22], and prolonged administration of antiemetics of short plasma half-life (at least until 12 hours after i.v. CMF) has been recommended [22].

In a randomised study performed by Chiara et al. [23] in 68 i.v. CMF-treated patients, intravenous methylprednisolone administered in either 375 mg or 120 mg doses divided into 3 parts was able to provide complete emetic control during the 24 hours after chemotherapy in 66% and 71% of the patients, respectively.

Ondansetron (8 mg per os before chemotherapy and then 8 mg tds for 3 to 5 days) was evaluated in a pilot study carried out in 29 patients treated with i.v. CMF [24]. In the first course of CMF, complete protection from vomiting was observed in 86% of patients. Nausea was absent in 62% of the cases in the same course.

High-dose dexamethasone (24 mg in 5 doses) has been proven to be superior to placebo and a single dose of i.v. metoclopramide (1 mg/kg) in the control of i.v. CMF-induced emesis [25].

Intravenous methylprednisolone (125 mg prior to i.v. CMF) was more effective than a single administration of low-dose metoclopramide (20 mg i.v. prior to chemotherapy), providing complete (no vomiting) and partial (1-2 vomiting episodes) protection in 11% and 63% of patients, respectively, versus 0% and 11% with metoclopramide [26]. A single dose of either low or high-dose metoclopramide, therefore, is not an appropriate antiemetic treatment for i.v. CMF-treated patients. However, metoclopramide administered in 5 intravenous doses of 20 mg every 3 hours was as effective as methylprednisolone (125 mg i.v. x 3 doses) in the control of i.v. CMF-induced emesis, with complete response rates of 76.5% and 66.7%, respectively [27]. The authors of this study suggested that the good results obtained with low-dose metoclopramide could be due to the intravenous administration of the drug every 3 hours for a prolonged period of time (up to 11.5 hours after chemotherapy), which allows for the control of the late vomiting usually seen with i.v. CMF.

The importance of the route and timing of administration of metoclopramide in the control of i.v. CMF-induced emesis was also made evident in a controlled study by Campora et al. [28]. In this trial, methylprednisolone (125 mg i.v. prior to CMF and 125 mg i.m. 6 and 12 hours after chemotherapy) was superior to metoclopramide (0.33 mg/kg i.v. prior to CMF and 0.33 mg/kg i.m. 6 and 12 hours later). Complete protection was observed in 58% of patients receiving methylprednisolone versus 20% of patients treated with metoclopramide. The poor results obtained with i.v. followed by i.m. metoclopramide in this study are in contrast with the results obtained by Roila et al. [27] using 5 doses of 20 mg of the drug administered intravenously every 3 hours. The route and timing of administration of metoclopramide seem to be of the utmost importance to obtain the maximum antiemetic benefit.

Silvey et al. [29] compared the antiemetic effectiveness of haloperidol plus dexamethasone versus prochlorperazine plus dexamethasone in breast cancer patients receiving FAC or i.v. CMF. All antiemetics were given as an initial intravenous dose (haloperidol 2 mg/m^2, prochlorperazine 6 mg/m^2, dexamethasone 5 mg/m^2) followed by the same dose orally every 4 hours for 24 hours. There was no significant difference between the two antiemetic regimens in the incidence of nausea and vomiting. Overall, 17 of the 24 CMF-treated patients (71%) obtained complete protection from vomiting and 14 (58%) had no nausea during the 24-hour study period.

A recent uncontrolled study assessed the antiemetic efficacy of the combination of methylprednisolone (80 mg i.v. prior to chemotherapy) plus the dopamine D_2 receptor antagonist thyethylperazine (6.5 mg per os prior to chemotherapy and 6.5 mg per os ever 8 hours for 3 days) in 31 women receiving 6 courses of i.v. CMF as adjuvant therapy for breast cancer [30]. The complete response rate at the first course was 90%. Sixty-eight percent of patients were free of emesis with this antiemetic combination all through the 6 scheduled courses of CMF chemotherapy.

In conclusion, the optimal antiemetic treatment for i.v. CMF chemotherapy has not yet been defined. Metoclopramide, corticoids and ondansetron seem to be moderately to highly effective in the control of i.v CMF-induced emesis. Metoclopramide is not very appropriate for outpatients because the drug has to be administered intravenously over prolonged periods of time. Ondansetron is safe and effective in the control of i.v. CMF-induced emesis, but its cost is an important concern in patients treated with moderately emetogenic chemotherapy that could be properly managed with less expensive antiemetic treatments. Methylprednisolone and dexamethasone seem more appropriate than metoclopramide for outpatients, but they provide complete emetic control in only 40-50% of i.v. CMF-treated patients. The combination of a corticoid and a D_2 dopamine antagonist merits further controlled evaluation in i.v. CMF-induced emesis.

Cyclophosphamide-Anthracycline Containing Combinations

Cyclophosphamide and doxorubicin or epirubicin are frequently associated in the treatment of breast cancer, often together with 5-fluorouracil (FAC, FEC, AC and EC regimens). These combinations are a frequent cause of emesis. Cyclophosphamide and doxorubicin/epirubicin are the main emetic stimuli of the combinations, while the contribution of 5-fluorouracil is of minor importance.

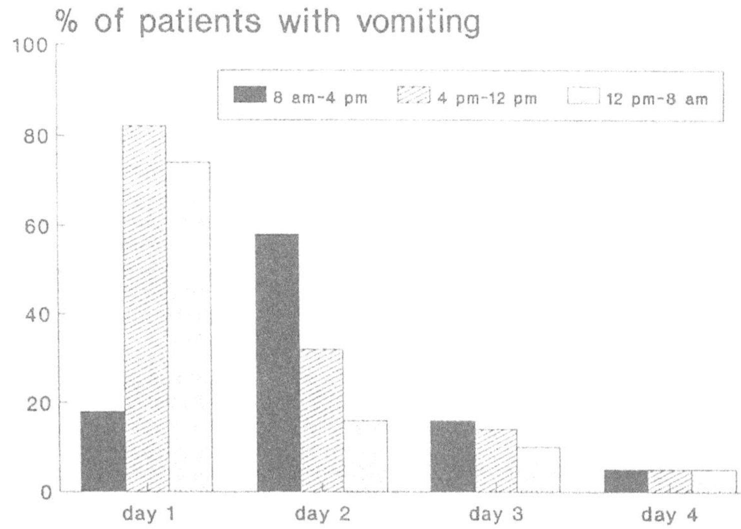

Fig. 1. The spontaneous course of FAC-induced emesis. Incidence of vomiting in breast cancer patients treated with FAC without antiemetic prophylaxis over 8-hour periods. FAC chemotherapy was administered over 1 hour starting between 11:00 and 12:00 a.m. on day 1. Reproduced from reference 31, with permission of the publisher

The FAC combination (5-fluorouracil 500 mg/m^2 i.v., doxorubicin 50 mg/m^2 i.v., cyclophosphamide 500 mg/m^2 i.v.) is widely used as adjuvant or palliative treatment for breast cancer. FAC is a severely emetogenic regimen. In a prospective evaluation carried out in 1982 in 31 patients who did not receive any antiemetic prophylaxis, 93.5% had one or more vomiting episodes during the first course of FAC chemotherapy [31]. The median number of emetic episodes was 16 and 74% of patients had 7 or more vomiting and/or retching episodes after the first course of FAC chemotherapy. The emetic time frame of FAC-induced emesis was also determined in this patient population (Fig. 1). Vomiting started after a median latency time of 5.5 hours. The median duration of vomiting was 17 hours (range: 0-84 hours). More than 50% of patients presented vomiting on the second day, but the emetic symptoms disappeared in the majority of patients on the third day.

The FEC combination (5-fluorouracil 500-600 mg i.v., epirubicin 50-75 mg/m^2 i.v., cyclophosphamide 500-600 mg/m^2 i.v.), widely used in Europe in substitution of the FAC regimen, is somewhat less emetogenic than FAC but still an important emetic challenge.

FAC is clearly more emetogenic than i.v. CMF [29], due to the additive emetic properties of cyclophosphamide and doxorubicin. The period of latency of vomiting with FAC chemotherapy is slightly shorter than with i.v. CMF, probably because of the doxorubicin contribution to emesis.

In spite of the fact that the combinations of cyclophosphamide and anthracyclines are widely used in the treatment of breast cancer, only a few trials have specifically addressed the control of emesis provoked by these combinations. Dopamine D_2 receptor antagonists and corticoids have been shown to be of limited value in the control of AC and FAC-induced emesis.

In a randomised, double-blind study on 29 patients receiving AC chemotherapy (doxorubicin 70 mg/m^2 plus cyclophosphamide 700 mg/m^2), Edge et al. [32] compared high-dose oral metoclopramide (2 mg/m^2 every 4 hours for 24 hours), high-dose intravenous metoclopramide (same dose) and prochlorperazine (10 mg orally every 4 hours for 24 hours). Statistical analysis showed no significant advantage of any regimen. The complete and major response rates on day 1 were 20%/60% (prochlorperazine), 30%/50% (oral metoclopramide) and 22%/22% (intravenous metoclopramide). Metoclopramide was poorly tolerated, with dystonic reactions in 32% of patients.

A randomised, double-blind, crossover study carried out by Diaz-Rubio et al. [33] in 46 women due to receive FAC chemotherapy, compared thyethylperazine (6.5 mg p.o. every 8 hours for 3 days) plus methylprednisolone (250 mg i.v. x 2 doses 2 hours apart) with thyethylperazine (same dose) plus placebo. The combination was clearly superior to thyethylperazine alone and was preferred by 70% of the patients. Complete and major (1-2 episodes) control of emesis with methylprednisolone plus thyethylperazine was achieved in 36% and 16% of patients, respectively, versus 18% and 9% with thyethylperazine alone.

The association of haloperidol plus dexamethasone was compared with prochlorperazine plus dexamethasone in a randomised study in patients receiving chemotherapy for breast cancer [29]. There was no statistically significant difference in the overall incidence of vomiting between the two arms. Nine of the 24 patients treated with FAC (37.5%) obtained complete protection from vomiting and 5 (21%) were free of nausea with the antiemetic combinations.

The antiemetic effectiveness of the combination of i.v. methylprednisolone (250 mg prior to chemotherapy) plus oral thyethylperazine (6.5 mg every 8 hours for 3 days) and amitriptyline (25 mg every 8 hours for 3 days) was assessed in 107 breast cancer patients due to receive 6 courses of adjuvant FAC chemotherapy [34]. The complete response rate was 63% at the first course. However, a gradual decrease in complete protection rate was evident during the 6 courses of FAC chemotherapy, with only 49% of 107 patients free of vomiting after the sixth course.

A multicentre crossover trial compared methylprednisolone (120 mg i.v.) with beta-1-24 ACTH (0.5 mg i.m.) in 94 patients treated with FEC chemotherapy [36]. Both drugs were of similar efficacy. At the first course, no vomiting was observed in 51% of the patients treated with ACTH versus 64% with methylprednisolone.

The antiemetic activity of the antiserotoninergic ondansetron has been studied in a few studies on patients treated with cyclophosphamide-anthracycline combinations. Fraschini et al. [36] assessed the efficacy of 3 different dose levels of ondansetron (1 mg, 4 mg and 8 mg) given orally 3 times a day in patients receiving cyclophosphamide-doxorubicin based chemotherapy. No emesis was observed during the 2-day study period in 85% of patients treated with the 8 mg dose, 65% of patients treated with 4 mg and 55% of patients treated with 1 mg.

Bonneterre et al. [37] compared metoclopramide and ondansetron in 75 breast cancer patients scheduled to receive FAC or FEC chemotherapy. Antiemetics were given as a loading dose (metoclopramide, 60 mg i.v. plus 20 mg orally before chemotherapy; ondansetron, 4 mg i.v. plus 4 mg orally before chemotherapy) followed by oral doses every 8 hours for up to 3 days (metoclopramide 20 mg, ondansetron 8 mg). Ondansetron was significantly superior to metoclopramide in the control of emesis on day 1 and on days 2-3. On day 1, 66% of patients treated with ondansetron were complete responders versus 27% with metoclopramide. On days 2 and 3, the complete protection rate with ondansetron dropped to 58%.

Ondansetron and metoclopramide were compared in another, similar study on patients treated with cyclophosphamide-doxorubicin or cyclophosphamide-epirubicin combinations [38]. Ondansetron was given as an initial intravenous infusion of 8 mg followed by 8 mg orally 3 times daily for up to 5 days. Metoclopramide was administered as an intravenous loading dose of 60 mg followed by 20 mg orally 3 times a day also for up to 5 days. Ninety-three patients (74 women, 19 men) entered the study. Complete antiemetic protection in the 24 hours following chemotherapy was observed in 65% of patients receiving ondansetron and in 41% of patients receiving metoclopramide, a statistically significant difference. The complete protection from vomiting on the worst of the 3 days following chemotherapy also favoured ondansetron (52.5% versus 31%).

Two different dosages of oral ondansetron (8 mg twice versus 3 times daily for 3 days) following a single intravenous dose of 8 mg of the antiemetic were compared in a randomised study in patients treated with cyclophosphamide-anthracycline containing combinations [39]. Both schedules were equally effective in controlling nausea and emesis. The twice-daily oral treatment prevented emesis in 65% of patients over 3 days after chemotherapy.

Campora et al. [40] compared the combinations of ondansetron (8 mg 3 times daily for 3 days) plus dexamethasone (20 mg i.v. prior to chemotherapy) versus metoclopramide (3 mg/kg i.v. x 2 doses followed by oral administration over 3 days) plus dexamethasone (20 mg i.v. prior to chemotherapy followed by 8 mg i.m. bid for 3 days) in 64 female chemotherapy-naive patients scheduled to receive FEC or FAC chemotherapy. Seventy-four percent of patients treated with the ondansetron combination did not vomit during the first 24 hours, compared with 43% receiving the metoclopramide combination. The worst-day analysis on days 2 to 5 showed 65% complete protection with the ondansetron combination versus 43% with metoclopramide-dexamethasone.

In conclusion, the combination of i.v. cyclophosphamide plus doxorubicin or epirubicin is severely emetogenic. Dopamine D_2 receptor antagonists and corticoids, alone or in combination, are of limited value in the control of emesis induced by this chemotherapy. Antiserotoninergic agents seem to be the antiemetic treatment of choice for patients receiving these combinations. The optimal duration of antiemetic treatment needs to be determined in appropriate studies, but 2 to 3 days could be a reasonable choice, taking into consideration the emetic time frame of cyclophosphamide-anthracycline containing combinations. At present there is no reason for the use of different schedules of antiemetics for the acute and delayed phases of emesis in patients receiving cyclophosphamide plus anthracyclines.

The addition of a corticoid to the 5-HT_3 receptor antagonist seems logical, since nearly one-third of patients treated with ondansetron alone did not obtain complete protection from emesis. However, the definitive interest of such an association should be demonstrated in prospective, randomised trials carried out in the specific population of patients treated with cyclophosphamide-anthracycline combinations.

Carboplatin

Carboplatin is currently used in the treatment of ovarian carcinoma (usually in combination with cyclophosphamide) and small-cell lung cancer (in combination with etoposide). This second-generation platinum analogue induces a specific pattern of emesis, which is characterised by a late onset of vomiting (more than 6 hours) [6]. Carboplatin provokes nausea and vomiting in more than 80% of patients when prophylactic antiemetics are not routinely used [6]. Nevertheless, only a few trials have addressed the specific issue of the control of carboplatin-induced emesis. In a pilot study [41], 25 patients who had presented 3 or more vomiting episodes with carboplatin in the previous course in spite of the use of conventional antiemetic regimens (mainly high-dose metoclopramide-dexamethasone combinations), were treated with ondansetron (8 mg p.o. before carboplatin and 8 mg p.o. every 8 hours for 5 days). Seventeen patients (68%) were completely free of vomiting during the first 24 hours after carboplatin and 14 patients (56%) for the full 5-day study period. Twenty-three of the patients vomited less than on their previous course with standard antiemetics and 22 of them chose to receive ondansetron in subsequent courses of carboplatin.

Smith et al. [10] reported the antiemetic control achieved with ondansetron in 34 ovarian cancer patients who were receiving carboplatin (400 mg/m^2). Ondansetron was given as 4 mg oral plus 4 mg intravenous 30 minutes prior to carboplatin followed by 8 mg p.o every 8 hours for 5 days. For the 5-day period as a whole, 65% of 18 previously untreated patients and 46% of 16 patients refractory to conventional antiemetics reported complete control of nausea and vomiting. The authors conclude that ondansetron is higly effective in controlling carboplatin-induced emesis and suggest that 3 days of oral therapy should be sufficient for the control of emesis.

Gridelli et al. [42] assessed the antiemetic efficacy of ondansetron (8 mg orally prior to chemotherapy, followed by 8 mg orally twice a day for 5 days) in 15 chemotherapy-naive cancer patients due to receive carboplatin (300 mg/m^2) in combination with other cytostatics (cyclophosphamide, epirubicin, 5-fluorouracil, vindesine). Fifteen patients (75%) obtained complete control of emesis in the first 24 hours after chemotherapy. Although the authors stated that the efficacy of ondansetron in the prevention of delayed carboplatin-induced emesis was unclear, all patients who achieved complete control in the acute phase (75%) obtained a similar control on days 2 to 5.

In a single-blind, randomised, parallel-group study, carried out in patients due to receive several moderately emetogenic chemotherapy regimens, granisetron (40 µg/kg i.v. prior to chemotherapy) was compared with chlorpromazine plus dexamethasone [17]. Overall, 24-hour efficacy was significantly higher in the granisetron group (68% complete response versus 47% in the comparator group). In the subset of patients treated with carboplatin (300 mg/m^2 or more, n = 78 patients), 65% of granisetron-treated patients and 23% of patients receiving chlorpromazine plus dexamethasone obtained a complete response during the first 24 hours. Unfortunately, the complete response rate over the 5-day period after carboplatin was not specifically reported.

These data suggest that a 5-HT_3 antagonist is probably indicated as first-line antiemetic treatment in patients treated with carboplatin, especially in female patients receiving carboplatin in combination with cyclophosphamide, since this population is at high risk of emesis with other antiemetics. Ondansetron or granisetron do not control emesis in the totality of carboplatin-treated patients, therefore the association of antiserotoninergics with corticosteroids should be tested in randomised prospective trials. Although the optimal duration of antiemetic treatment needs to be determined in appropriate studies, 2 to 3 days could be a reasonable choice, taking into consideration the emetic time frame of carboplatin.

Dacarbazine (DTIC)

Dacarbazine is one of the most emetogenic of chemotherapeutic agents. Virtually all patients treated with standard doses (250 mg/m^2 daily for 5 days or 800 to 1200 mg/m^2 in a single dose) experience nausea and vomiting. Dacarbazine-induced emesis is so severe that it has been considered one of the dose-limiting toxicities of the drug. The agent is usually administered in a 5-day schedule in order to decrease the emetic toxicity. With this fractionated administration, tolerance to its emetic effect in the last 2-3 days of therapy has been described.

The emetic time frame of dacarbazine-induced emesis is characterised by an early onset of vomiting (1-3 hours) and a short duration of emesis (usually less than 12 hours) [14].

Only a few studies in the literature have provided data on the control of dacarbazine-induced emesis. Tyson et al. [43] treated 10 patients receiving single-dose dacarbazine (1000 mg/m^2) with high-dose metoclopramide (2 mg/kg i.v. 30 minutes before dacarbazine and 2 mg/kg i.v. every 2 hours for 4 doses). Seven of the patients had not previously received chemotherapy. Four patients (40%) obtained complete control of emesis over the 24-hour study period and 5 additional patients had major control (1-2 emetic episodes).

Basurto et al. [44] compared the efficacy and tolerability of high-dose i.v. metoclopramide (2 mg/kg x 4 doses) versus metoclopramide plus high-dose i.v. methylprednisolone (250 mg x 2 doses) in 34 patients treated with dacarbazine (250 mg/m^2/day x 5 days) alone or in combination with cyclophosphamide, doxorubicin and vincristine. The antiemetics were given only on the first 2 days of chemotherapy since tolerance to the emetic effect of dacarbazine was expected in the following days. The combination was slightly superior to metoclopramide alone only on the second day of chemotherapy. Nearly 75% of patients obtained complete control of emesis in the first two days of chemotherapy. Thirteen of the 32 evaluable patients (47%) did not vomit during the 5 days of chemotherapy. There was a relapse of vomiting in nearly one-third of patients after the discontinuation of antiemetics. Extrapyramidal reactions increased significantly from the first day (6%) to the second day (26%), probably due to the cumulative toxicity of metoclopramide.

Smith and the Granisetron Study Group [12] compared 2 dose levels of granisetron (40 and 160 μg/kg) in patients receiving moderately emetogenic chemotherapy. Overall, no differences in efficacy or safety between the two doses were observed. In 28 dacarbazine-treated patients (300-500 mg/m^2), the complete response rate over the first 24 hours approached 80%.

At present antiserotoninergics, alone or perhaps in combination with corticoids, seem to be a reasonable choice for the control of emesis in dacarbazine-treated patients. The minimum duration of antiemetic treatment for DTIC-treated patients (1 versus 2 or more days) needs to be determined in prospective studies.

Other Cytotoxic Agents

The efficacy of the uroprotector mesna in controlling haemorrhagic cystitis, one of the dose-limiting toxicities of the cyclophosphamide analogue ifosfamide, allows the administration of relatively high doses of this cytotoxic (4-10 g/m^2) over 1 to 5 days. At such high doses, ifosfamide provokes emesis in the majority of patients. A single pilot study has reported on the control of ifosfamide-induced emesis with the antiserotoninergic ondansetron [45]. Six patients receiving 4-6 g/m^2 of ifosfamide over 24 hours, in whom high-dose metoclopramide had failed to control the emesis in previous ifosfamide courses, were given 8 mg of ondansetron every 6 hours for 4 doses. Major control (0-2 emetic episodes) was observed in 4 patients. Six additional chemotherapy-naive patients receiving their first course of ifosfamide (same dose) were given 4 mg of ondansetron every 6 hours. Major emetic control was reached in 5 of the 6 patients.

Antiemetic studies addressing the control of vomiting induced by anthracyclines as the main emetogenic stimulus are scarce, probably because these agents are usually combined with cyclophosphamide (see above). Donati et al. [46] performed a controlled study of two different doses of methylprednisolone (125 mg or 40 mg i.v. before chemotherapy and the same dose 6 and 12 hours later) in 30 outpatients receiving epirubicin (50 mg/m^2 or more) alone or in combination with other cytotoxics. Both doses had similar effectiveness, with complete control of emesis in over 50% of patients.

Fluorouracil is widely used in the treatment of colorectal cancer, often as a single drug. The classic schedule of administration (daily bolus x 5 days) has progressively been substituted by more sophisticated regimens (high-dose continuous infusion, weekly administration, etc.). In recent years, fluorouracil has been associated with the biomodulator leucovorin in order to potentiate its antitumoral activity. Leucovorin does not seem to have emetic properties. Fluorouracil is classically considered to belong to the group of cytotoxics of low emetic potential. Nevertheless, placebo-controlled studies have shown that 80% and 44% of 5-FU-treated patients, respectively, present nausea and vomiting, usually of slight to mild intensity [47]. In two historical trials, Moertel et al. [47,48] demonstrated for the first time the effectiveness of several oral phenothiazines (prochlorperazine, thiopropazate, thyethylperazine) in the control of fluorouracil-induced emesis. Phenothiazines provided complete control of vomiting in 75-80% of patients receiving bolus administration of fluorouracil.

Methotrexate is scarcely emetogenic when used in conventional doses (40 to 60 mg/m^2 i.v.). However, a single study has reported that high-dose methotrexate (6-12 g/m^2) administered with leucovorin calcium rescue induces nausea and vomiting in 72% of placebo-treated patients [49]. In this study, thetrahydrocannabinol was able to reduce the incidence, severity and duration of nausea and vomiting provoked by high-dose methotrexate, providing complete control of vomiting over several courses of chemotherapy in nearly 40% of patients.

Nausea and vomiting have been reported in virtually all patients treated with high-dose cytosine arabinoside. Craig et al. [50] studied the activity of high-dose metoclopramide (2 mg/kg every 2 hours x 4 doses) in the control of high-dose cytosine arabinoside-induced emesis in 33 haematologic patients. Fifty-one percent of patients had complete control of vomiting and 18% presented only 1 or 2 emetic episodes. However, grade 2 nausea was almost universal (32 of 33 patients) despite metoclopramide.

Acute Versus Delayed Emesis in Moderately Emetogenic Chemotherapy

In spite of the lack of evidence that acute (first 24 hours) and delayed (days 2 to 5) emesis after non-cisplatin containing combinations have different pathogenetic mechanisms, many large trials have reported the control of emesis separately in these two periods of time. We would like to comment on two of the most important of these trials, in order to show the interest and limitations of such an approach. Jones et al. [13] compared ondansetron and dexamethasone given over 5 days for the prophylaxis of acute and delayed emesis and nausea induced by moderately emetogenic chemotherapy. Details on the chemotherapeutic regimens and doses received by the patients were not provided, but "most patients received a combination chemotherapy regimen including an intravenous anthracycline, and/or cyclophosphamide, and/or etoposide". The study, carried out during 2 consecutive cycles with the same chemotherapy, was multicentre, randomised, double-blind and crossover. Patients taking ondansetron or dexamethasone reported no significant differences in complete and major control of acute (83% versus 79%, p = 0.46) or delayed (82% versus 88%, p = 0.214) vomiting. Significantly more patients on dexamethasone (87%) than on ondansetron (72%) reported control of delayed nausea (days 2-5), but the real meaning of this fact is controversial since patients reported a similar preference for ondansetron (40%) and dexamethasone (30%) after the second course of chemotherapy. The authors concluded that ondansetron and dexamethasone offer an adequate outpatient control of chemotherapy-induced emesis, although dexamethasone has an advantage in the control of delayed nausea. A relevant point in this study is the evidence that ondansetron and dexamethasone were effective in both the acute and the delayed phases of emesis induced by non-cisplatin containing chemotherapy, thus suggesting a common mechanism of emesis in both phases, in contrast with cisplatin-induced emesis. Since 5-HT_3 antagonists and corticoids possess different mechanisms of control of emesis, the combination of both drugs appears to be a reasonable approach for the control of emesis induced by non-cisplatin containing chemotherapy. The Italian Group for Antiemetic Research tested this hypothesis in a randomised study involving 428 patients who were to receive non-cisplatin containing chemotherapy (cyclophosphamide 600-1000 mg/m^2, doxorubicin 50 or more mg/m^2, epirubicin 75 or more mg/m^2 or carboplatin 300 or more mg/m^2, either alone or in some combination) [51]. Patients were randomised to receive either granisetron (a single i.v. dose of 3 mg before chemotherapy), dexamethasone (8 mg i.v. before chemotherapy, 4 mg p.o. before chemotherapy and 4 mg p.o. at 6, 12, and 18 hours afterwards) or the combination of both drugs. In the first 24 hours, complete protection from vomiting and nausea was achieved in 70.6% and 55.1%, respectively, of the patients receiving dexamethasone, in 72.3% and 48.2% of the patients receiving granisetron, and in 92.6% and 71.9% of the patients receiving granisetron plus dexamethasone ($p<0.001$ for all comparisons). Patients who received granisetron alone had less protection from delayed vomiting (day 2) and delayed nausea (days 2-3) than those who received dexamethasone alone or the combination of granisetron and dexamethasone. The authors concluded that granisetron combined with dexamethasone is the most effective regimen for the prevention of emesis induced by moderately emetogenic chemotherapy. The two arms containing dexamethasone were more effective in the control of nausea and vomiting on days 2-3, but this finding may be explained by the fact that granisetron was only given before chemotherapy, while the last dose of dexamethasone was given 18 hours afterwards. This study clearly showed that the combination of a 5-HT_3 antagonist plus dexamethasone is the best antiemetic treatment for the first 24 hours in patients treated with non-cisplatin containing chemotherapy. The best antiemetic approach for days 2 to 5 must be determined in a new study in which patients receiving granisetron plus dexamethasone on the first day are randomised to receive either granisetron, dexamethasone or the combination of both on days 2 to 5.

Conclusive Remarks

The progress made in the control of emesis induced by non-cisplatin-containing regimens in the past decade has been remarkable. We have obtained a considerable amount of information about the characteristics of the emesis provoked by many chemotherapeutic drugs and their combinations and we have identified many of the problems we need to deal with. In addition, the antiemetic armamentarium has been extraordinarily reinforced with new, very active antiemetics, such as the antiserotoninergic drugs. The methodology of antiemetic trials has also clearly improved. Yet, when the clinician tries to find in the literature clear guidelines for the management of some specific emetic situations, many gaps become evident. At present we have clear ideas about the achievements and limitations in the control of acute and delayed cisplatin-induced emesis, but we lack similar information for a number of non-cisplatin containing combinations. Unfortunately, it has become evident that the extrapolation and generalisation of conclusions from antiemetic trials conducted in cisplatin-treated patients to other populations has many limitations, as discussed elsewhere [7]. More regimen-specific antiemetic trials are required that aim at providing practical and concrete guidelines for the emetic control in particular subsets of patients (e.g. female patients treated with FAC chemotherapy), rather than general studies carried out in miscellaneous patient populations [30]. We are confident that the current trend to perform such regimen-specific antiemetic trials will allow us to produce, in the near future, an updated version of this chapter containing more precise guidelines for the management of emesis induced by cytotoxic agents different from cisplatin.

REFERENCES

1 Pater JL, Willan AR: Methodologic issues in trials of antiemetics. J Clin Oncol 1984 (2):484-487
2 Tonato M, Roila F, Del Favero A: Methodology of antiemetic trials: A review. Ann Oncol 1991 (2):107-114
3 Kris MG, Gralla RJ, Clark RA et al: Incidence, course and severity of delayed nausea and vomiting following the administration of high-dose cisplatin. J Clin Oncol 1985 (3):1379-1384
4 Gandara DR, Harvey WH, Monaghan GG, Perez EA, Hesketh PJ: Delayed emesis following high-dose cisplatin: a double-blind randomized comparative trial of ondansetron (GR38032F) versus placebo. Eur J Cancer 1993 (29A Suppl 1):S35-S38
5 Fetting JH, Grochow LB, Folstein MF, Ettinger DS, Colvin M: The course of nausea and vomiting after high-dose cyclophosphamide. Cancer Treat Rep 1982 (66):1487-1493
6 Martin M, Diaz-Rubio E, Sanchez A, Almenarez J, Lopez-Vega JM: The natural course of emesis after carboplatin treatment. Acta Oncol 1990 (29):593-595
7 Martin M: Myths and realities of antiemetic treatment. Br J Cancer 1992 (66 Suppl XIX):S46-S51
8 Rosso R, Campora E, Cetto G, Fosser V, Marangolo M, Oliva C: Oral ondansetron for the control of acute and delayed cyclophosphamide-induced emesis. Anticancer Res 1991 (11):937-939
9 Schmoll HJ: The role of ondansetron in the treatment of emesis induced by non-cisplatin containing chemotherapy regimens. Eur J Cancer Clin Oncol 1989 (25 Suppl 1):S35-S39
10 Smith DB, Rustin GJ, Howells N, Lambert HE, McQuade B: A phase II study of ondansetron as antiemetic prophylaxis in patients receiving carboplatin for advanced ovarian cancer. Ann Oncol 1991 (2):607-608
11 Warr D, Willan A, Fine S et al: Superiority of granisetron to dexamethasone plus prochlorperazine in the prevention of chemotherapy-induced emesis. JNCI 1991 (83):1169-1173
12 Smith IE on behalf of the Granisetron Study Group: A comparison of two dose levels of granisetron in patients receiving moderately emetogenic cytostatic chemotherapy. Eur J Cancer 1990 (26 Suppl 1):S19-S22
13 Jones AL, Hill AS, Soukop M et al: Comparison of dexamethasone and ondansetron in the prophylaxis of emesis induced by moderately emetogenic chemotherapy. Lancet 1991 (338):483-487
14 Borison HL, McCarthy LE: Neuropharmacology of chemotherapy-induced emesis. Drugs 1993 (25 Suppl 1):8-17
15 Cubeddu LX, Hoffman IS, Fuenmayor NT, Finn AL: Antagonism of serotonin S-3 receptors with ondansetron prevents nausea and emesis induced by cyclophosphamide-containing chemotherapy regimens. J Clin Oncol 1990 (8):1721-1727
16 Herrstedt J, Sigsgaard T, Boesgaard M, Jensen TP, Dombernofsky P: Ondansetron plus metopimazine compared with ondansetron alone in patients receiving moderately emetogenic chemotherapy. N Engl J Med 1993 (328):1076-1080
17 Marty M on behalf of the Granisetron Study Group: A comparison of granisetron as a single agent with conventional combination antiemetic therapies in the treatment of cytostatic-induced emesis. Eur J Cancer 1992 (28A Suppl 1):S12-S16
18 Morrow GR, Loughner JE, Bennet JM: Prevalence of nausea and vomiting and other side effects in patients receiving cytoxan, methotrexate, fluorouracil (CMF) therapy with and without prednisone. Proc ASCO 1984 (3):105
19 Buser K, Joss R, Piquet D et al: A randomized, double-blind comparison of oral ondansetron and placebo in the prophylaxis of CMF-induced nausea and vomiting. Proc ASCO 1990 (9):331
20 Levitt M, Warr D, Yelle L et al: Ondansetron compared with dexamethasone and metoclopramide as antiemetics in the chemotherapy of breast cancer with cyclophosphamide, methotrexate, and 5-fluorouracil. N Engl J Med 1993 (328):1081-1084
21 David M, Durand M, Chauvergne J, Mauriac L, Bui BN, Hoerni B: Cyclophosphamide, methotrexate, and 5-FU (CMF)-induced nausea and vomiting: A controlled study with high-dose metoclopramide. Cancer Treat Rep 1984 (68):921-922
22 Roila F, Minotti V, Ballatori E, Basurto C, Tonato M: Evaluation of the antiemetic activity of bromopride in cancer patients treated with i.v. CMF. Tumori 1985 (71):455-458
23 Chiara S, Campora E, Lionetto R, Bruzzi P, Rosso R: Methylprednisolone for the control of CMF-induced emesis. Am J Clin Oncol 1987 (10):264-267
24 Campora E, Oliva C, Mammoliti S et al: Oral ondansetron (GR 38032F) for the control of CMF-induced emesis in the outpatient. Breast Cancer Res Treat 1991 (19): 129-132
25 Pollera CF, Nardi M, Marolla P, Pinaro P, Terzoli E, Giannarelli D: Effective control of CMF-related emesis with high-dose dexamethasone: results of a double-blind crossover trial with metoclopramide and placebo. Am J Clin Oncol 1989 (12):524-529
26 Gez E, Sulkes A, Ochayon L et al: Methylprednisolone versus metoclopramide as antiemetic treatment in patients receiving adjuvant cyclophosphamide, methotrexate, 5-fluorouracil (CMF) chemotherapy: A randomized crossover blind study. J Chemother 1989 (1):365-368
27 Roila F, Basurto C, Minotti V, Ballatori E, Tonato M, Del Favero A: Methylprednisolone versus metoclopramide for prevention of nausea and vomiting in breast cancer patients treated with intravenous cyclophosphamide, methotrexate, 5-fluorouracil: A double-blind, randomized study. Oncology 1988 (45):346-349
28 Campora E, Chiara S, Bruzzi P, Scarsi P, Rosso R: The antiemetic efficacy of methylprednisolone compared with metoclopramide in outpatients receiving adjuvant CMF chemotherapy for breast cancer: A randomized trial. Tumori 1985 (71):459-462
29 Silvey L, Carpenter JT, Wheeler RH, Lee J, Conolley C: A randomized comparison of haloperidol plus dexamethasone versus prochlorperazine plus dexamethasone in preventing nausea and vomiting in patients receiving chemotherapy for breast cancer. J Clin Oncol 1988 (6):1397-1400

30 Martin M, Aranda E, Diaz-Rubio E et al: Emetic control in breast cancer patients receiving i.v. CMF: Results of two consecutive studies using a new method of assessment. Oncology Rep 1996 (3): 115-121

31 Martin Jimenez M, Diaz-Rubio E, Blazquez Encinar JC et al: Tolerancia, toxicidad y aceptación del tratamiento quimioterápico FAC (5-fluorouracilo, adriamicina y ciclofosfamida) en el cáncer de mama. Análisis de 100 pacientes consecutivas. Neoplasia 1988 (5):8-14

32 Edge SB, Funkhouser WK, Berman A et al: High-dose oral and intravenous metoclopramide in doxorubicin/cyclophosphamide-induced emesis. Am J Clin Oncol 1987 (10):257-263

33 Diaz-Rubio E, Martin M, Rosell R, Valerdi JJ, Gonzalez-Larriba JL, Barriga JJ: The antiemetic efficacy of thyethylperazine and methylprednisolone versus thyethylperazine and placebo in breast cancer patients treated with adjuvant chemotherapy (fluorouracil, doxorubicin, and cyclophosphamide). A randomized, double-blind, cross-over trial. Acta Oncologica 1991 (30):339-342

34 Martin M, Diaz-Rubio E, Casado A, Dominguez S, Sastre J: Progressive loss of antiemetic efficacy during subsequent courses of chemotherapy. Eur J Cancer 1992 (28):430-432

35 Bonneterre J, Kerbrat P, Fargeot P et al: A multicenter randomized cross-over trial comparing methylprednisolone (120 mg, IV) to beta-1-24 ACTH (0.5 mg, IM) in the prophylaxis of emesis induced by FEC regimen. Proc ASCO 1990 (9):1231

36 Fraschini G, Ciociola A, Esparza L et al: Evaluation of three oral dosages of ondansetron in the prevention of nausea and emesis associated with cyclophosphamide-doxorubicin chemotherapy. J Clin Oncol 1991 (9):1268-1274

37 Bonneterre J, Chevalier B, Metz R et al: A randomized double-blind comparison of ondansetron and metoclopramide in the prophylaxis of emesis induced by cyclophosphamide, fluorouracil and doxorubicin or epirubicin chemotherapy. J Clin Oncol 1990 (8):1063-1069

38 Kaasa S, Kvaloy S, Dicato MA et al: A comparison of ondansetron with metoclopramide in the prophylaxis of chemotherapy-induced nausea and vomiting: A randomized, double-blind study. Eur J Cancer 1990 (26):311-314

39 Dicato MA, Kaasa S, Campora E et al: Efficacy of twice daily versus three times daily oral ondansetron in the prevention of chemotherapy-induced emesis: A randomized, single-blind, multicentre study. The Ondansetron International Study Group. Clin Oncol (R Coll Radiol) 1992 (4):275-279

40 Campora E, Giudici S, Merlini L, Rosso R: Control of acute, delayed FEC/FAC-induced emesis and GI toxicity at subsequent cycles: A randomized trial of metoclopramide, dexamethasone and orphenadrine vs ondansetron and dexamethasone. Proc ASCO 1992 (11):1358

41 Harvey VJ, Evans BD, Mitchell PLR et al: Reduction of carboplatin induced emesis by ondansetron. Br J Cancer 1991 (63):942-944

42 Gridelli C, Incoronato P, Airona G, Pepe R, Arpinelli F, Bianco AR: Ondansetron in the prophylaxis of nausea and vomiting induced by carboplatin combination chemotherapy. Eur J Cancer 1993 (29A):651

43 Tyson LB, Clark RA, Gralla RJ: High-dose metoclopramide: Control of dacarbazine-induced emesis in a preliminary trial. Cancer Treat Rep 1982 (66): 2108

44 Basurto C, Roila F, Tonato M, Ballatori E, Buzzi F, Calabresi F, Del Favero A: Antiemetic activity of high-dose metoclopramide combined with methylprednisolone versus metoclopramide alone in dacarbazine-treated cancer patients. Am J Clin Oncol 1989 (12):235-238

45 Green JA, Watkin SW, Hammond P, Griggs, Challoner T: The efficacy and safety of GR38032F in the prophylaxis of ifosfamide induced nausea and vomiting. Cancer Chemother Pharmacol 1989 (23 Suppl):67

46 Dokati D, Gilli G, Indelli M, Marzola M, Santini A, Malacarne P: Methylprednisolone in control of 4'-epidoxorubicin-induced emesis. Proceedings ECCO-4 (Fourth European Conference on Clinical Oncology and Cancer Nursing). Madrid, November 1987 p 281

47 Moertel CG, Reitemeier RJ, Gage RP: A controlled clinical evaluation of antiemetic drugs. JAMA 1963 (186):116-118

48 Moertel CG, Reitemeier RJ: Controlled clinical studies of orally administered antiemetic drugs. Gastroenterology 1969 (57):262-268

49 Chang AE, Shiling DJ, Stillman RC et al: Dealta-9-tetrahydrocannabinol as an antiemetic in cancer patients receiving high-dose methotrexate. A prospective, randomized evaluation. Ann Intern Med 1979 (91):819-824

50 Craig JB, Powell BL, White DR, Capizzi RL: Antiemetic therapy in patients treated with high-dose cytosine arabinoside. Oncology 1987 (44):90-92

51 The Italian Group for Antiemetic Research: Dexamethasone, granisetron, or both for the prevention of nausea and vomiting during chemotherapy for cancer. N Engl J Med 1995 (332):1-5

Therapeutic Approach to Delayed Emesis

Matti S. Aapro

Divisione di Oncologia Medica, Istituto Europeo di Oncologia, via Ripamonti 435, 20141 Milano, Italy, and Division d'Onco-Hématologie, Hôpital Cantonal Universitaire, 1211 Genève, Switzerland

The remarkable progress in the control of cancer therapy-related emesis that we have witnessed over the past few years is well reflected in this monograph. At present, in adults submitted to highly emetogenic chemotherapy, nausea and vomiting should be a rare event in the first 24 hours of observation, with only 5% or less of the patients failing antiemetic therapy completely (more than 5 episodes of emesis), and over 60% fully protected from both nausea and vomiting. However, these figures conceal the reality: if one looks at the whole experience of the patient and includes the later days after chemotherapy in the observation period, the results are clearly not as favourable. Delayed emesis, defined as emesis or retching occurring after the first 24 hours of observation, is present in many patients and influences both the outcome of the acute phase of the next chemotherapy cycle and anticipatory emesis, a conditioned reflex which is very difficult to treat [1].

Physiology of Delayed Emesis

Unfortunately there is no animal model which allows the study of delayed emesis. Some models are in development, but today we have to admit that the ferret and the *Suncus murinus* are of use only in the evaluation of acute emesis, as described by Andrews in this volume. His group [2] has proposed several reasons for the onset of this phenomenon, which might not be related to serotonin release in the gut (Table 1). Cerebral oedema along with increased intracranial pressure is a common cause of nausea and vomiting, and since corticosteroids have a protective effect against delayed emesis and constitute the treatment of choice for cerebral oedema, one can speculate on this possible cause of delayed emesis. A more likely reason for delayed emesis is disordered gut function, through damage to the intestinal mucosa by the anticancer treatment. Also related to this damage are products of cell breakdown, and some evidence for this has been found by Andrews' group.

Table 1. Physiology of delayed emesis

* Serotonin has a minimal role
* Blood-brain barrier, cerebral oedema?
* Disturbed gut motility
* Cellular breakdown products

Clinical Observations: Causes of Delayed Emesis

Type and Dose of Chemotherapy

There is no doubt that very high-dose cisplatin-based chemotherapy is almost always followed by delayed emesis, in spite of the success of the initial antiemetic therapy. However, many chemotherapeutic agents are capable of inducing delayed emesis, and specifically cyclophosphamide - when used intravenously - and carboplatin can induce an incidence of delayed emesis which is well above 50% on days 2 to 7 after chemotherapy [3,4]. The role of the other drugs given concomitantly with these agents is not well defined, although it is accepted that combined chemotherapy is more emetogenic than single-agent therapy. The importance of the dose of cisplatin is the

Table 2. Determining the risk factors for delayed emesis

TYPE OF CHEMOTHERAPY AND DELAYED EMESIS	
• cisplatin > 49 mg/m^2:	22-50% incidence
• cisplatin > 90 mg/m^2:	43-89% incidence
• other combinations:	> 42% incidence
ACUTE CONTROL AND DELAYED EMESIS	
No acute emesis 26-47% incidence vs	absence of acute control 53-88% incidence
INFLUENCE OF SEX ON DELAYED EMESIS	
Male patients 39% incidence	Female patients 76% incidence
but acute phase control is also worse in females	

best described chemotherapy-related variable, with delayed phenomena appearing in 22% to 50% of the patients treated with cisplatin doses below 90 mg/m^2, while at higher doses the incidence is largely above those numbers, with figures from 43% to 89% reported in the literature [5-7] (Table 2).

Control in the First 24 Hours

It is understandable and has actually been observed that patients who experience no emesis in the first 24 hours after chemotherapy have a better control of nausea and vomiting in the subsequent days, compared to patients who do poorly initially. When patients receiving cisplatin-based chemotherapy achieve complete control on day 1, emesis in subsequent days is seen in 26-47%, while the incidence of emesis varies between 53% and 88% in patients who experienced prior vomiting [5-7, and Schneider M, data presented at the symposium "Advances in Emesis Control", 15th UICC, 1990]. These observations have been confirmed recently in a paper which discusses also the fact that the pattern of delayed emesis does not change in subsequent cycles, but clearly influences the success rate of acute emetic control at subsequent cycles [8].

Gender

It has been reported by several groups that in the acute phase of emetic control, female patients do worse than male patients. It is therefore difficult to evaluate whether the poor emetic control in females in the delayed phase is a real phenomenon or a carryover effect from the lack of control of day 1. Recent results failed to confirm that sex is a determinant of delayed emesis [8].

Treatment of Delayed Emesis

From the above considerations it is quite clear that delayed emesis depends on the control on day 1, and therefore all studies claiming that a better control of delayed emesis was observed with a certain drug have to control for day 1 efficacy. Furthermore, because of the variables described, non-controlled studies are of no use, as any claimed improvement may well be related to those variables only.

Corticosteroids

In a study on 60 patients undergoing cisplatin-based chemotherapy, ACTH was compared to placebo for 4 days following chemotherapy (with metoclopramide and dexamethasone administered on day 1). Patients on ACTH had a 43% incidence of delayed emesis, compared to 67% of those on placebo [9].
Some efficacy has been reported for dexamethasone (see Table 3), which reduces the

Table 3. "Classic" agents and delayed emesis. Studies on cisplatin-treated patients

Ref.	No. pts.	Acute phase	Delayed phase	CR rate	
[10]	60	iv mcp + dex	ACTH	57%	
			placebo	33%	
[7]	42	iv mcp + dex	same	75%	
			placebo	50%	
				N.	V.
[5]	120	iv mcp + dex	mcp 20 mg po qid	52%	69%
			dex 1 mg po qid	69%	65%
			placebo po qid	27%	57%
[6]	91	dex + met + lor	placebo	13%	
			dex 8 mg po qid	35%	
			dex + mcp 0.5 mg/kg po qid	52%	

mcp = metoclopramide; dex = dexamethasone; lor = lorazepam; N = nausea; V = vomiting; CR = complete response

incidence of delayed nausea [5] or emesis [7] in cisplatin-treated patients and of delayed emesis and nausea [10] in patients treated with moderately emetogenic chemotherapy. Dexamethasone, in delayed emesis too, potentiates metoclopramide, as detailed below.

Metoclopramide

Combinations of metoclopramide and dexamethasone have been for a long time the best acute antiemetic treatment, and the continuation of this intravenous combination over several days has decreased the incidence of emesis to 25% compared to 50% for placebo, in cisplatin-treated patients [7].

A protection from nausea of 52% is obtained with metoclopramide given orally at a dose of 20 mg 4 times a day for 7 days, versus 69% with dexamethasone 1 mg 4 times a day and 27% with placebo [5]. However, the incidence of emesis was 31%, 35% and 43%, respectively, thus limiting the value of either agent relative to that of placebo.

The last study comparing oral dexamethasone (8 mg 4 times/day for 2 days, then 4 mg 4 times/day for 2 days) with the same regimen plus oral metoclopramide (0.5 mg/kg 4 times/day for 4 days) and with placebo, has shown a clear superiority for the combination therapy [6] (Table 3).

5-HT$_3$ Receptor Antagonists

Although not a randomised comparison, the study by Kris et al. [11] which investigated the effectiveness of ondansetron against delayed emesis is of interest as it shows absolutely no effect of this agent in the delayed setting. Twenty patients treated initially with the same combination as used in their previous study [6] (see Table 3) had 15% complete protection from delayed emesis, a result similar to that previously reported with placebo.

Smyth reported at a Satellite of the 17th congress of the ESMO in Lyon, 1992, that in a study including 533 patients who were treated on day 1 with cisplatin and granisetron 40 µg/kg i.v., the use of oral granisetron at doses between 2.5 to 10 mg twice a day, on days 5 to 7 induced a 20% better complete protection rate in the granisetron arms compared to placebo; however, on days 2 to 4 the results were the same in all arms. Along the same lines is the study that looked at 0.5 mg of oral granisetron or 1.0 mg of oral granisetron both given twice daily and compared to placebo in 143 patients treated with high-dose cisplatin-based chemotherapy and 3 mg intravenous granisetron on day 1. Again, on days 4-6 after chemotherapy there seems to be an advantage for granisetron (especially the 1.0 b.d. group), but overall the complete protection rate is poor, with only 32% of the patients having no eme-

Table 4. 5-HT_3 antagonists and delayed emesis in moderately emetogenic chemotherapy

Ref.	No. pts.	Acute phase	Delayed phase	CR rate
[10]	112	ond 4 mg iv	ond 4 mg po qid	60%
		dex 8 mg iv	dex 4/1 po qid	72%
[14]	165	ond 8 mg po/tid	same	70%
		dex 10 mg iv	mcp 10 mg po tid	70%
[15]	301	dex + ond iv	ond 8 mg po bid	65%
		dex + ond iv	placebo	65%
		dex + ond iv	ond x 1 + placebo	45%

ond = ondansetron; mcp = metoclopramide; dex = dexamethasone; CR = complete response

sis from days 0 to 6 [data presented by P.H.M. de Mulder at an ESMO Satellite symposium, November 19, 1994].

Interestingly, patients who continued on metoclopramide 20 mg 3 times/day fared better (63% "complete and major responses") than patients on oral ondansetron 8 mg 3 times/day (56%) in a study where during the acute phase metoclopramide had been inferior (23% complete responses) to ondansetron (56% complete responses) [12].

A study [13] on 48 patients receiving cisplatin who had suffered from minimal emesis (up to 2 episodes) on day 1 shows somewhat better protection in the ondansetron arm, with response rates varying according to the type of analysis from 57% to 78% for ondansetron and 39-50% for placebo, failing to reach significance except on day 3 of follow-up. The study provides no details on patients' sex, type of chemotherapy and mean number of episodes of emesis in both arms, making any final conclusion impossible.

Table 4 summarizes several studies which have considered the possible role of serotonin antagonists for control of delayed emesis in the setting of moderately emetogenic chemotherapy. Studies on moderately emetogenic chemotherapy show no benefit for the arm with ondansetron [10,14,15]. It should be noted that we report the data of all 3 arms of the study of the NCIC [15] as presented at ASCO. Their final publication does not report the observations made in one of the arms because it did not have exactly the same antiemetic therapy on day 1; however, as it has been shown by others that a single dose of ondansetron may be equivalent to other modalities of administration, and the control rate on day 1 was actually the same in all 3 arms, we do not believe these data should be withheld.

There are no comparative data available to evaluate tropisetron in this setting, although the compound was developed for delayed-phase treatment. Data for dolasetron should be available soon, but there is little hope that it will be more encouraging.

Conclusion

Delayed emesis is far from being adequately understood or controlled. Furthermore, once we approach better control, it will be important to realise that in many instances delayed nausea and delayed vomiting are not the same phenomenon [16]. At present, the only recommendations are that one should avoid the use of serotonin-receptor antagonists in this setting, probably use a metoclopramide + dexamethasone or other dopamine antagonist with corticosteroid combination, and make sure patients do not irritate the gastrointestinal tract by overeating during the days after chemotherapy.

REFERENCES

1 Aapro MS, Kirchner V, Terrey JP: Anticipatory emesis: the role of granisetron. Br J Cancer 1994 (69): 957-960

2 Andrews PLR and Davis CJ: The mechanism of emesis induced by anti-cancer therapies. In: Andrews PLR and Sanger GJ: Emesis in Anti-Cancer Therapy: Mechanism and Treatment. Chapman & Hall, London 1993 pp 113-161

3 Martin M, Diaz-Rubio E, Sanchez A et al: The natural course of emesis after carboplatin treatment. Acta Oncologica 1990 (29):593-595

4 Aapro MS: 5-HT_3 receptor antagonists: an overview of their present status and future potential in cancer therapy-induced emesis. Drugs 1991 (42):551-586

5 Roila F, Boschetti E, Tonato M et al: Predictive factors of delayed emesis in cisplatin-treated patients and antiemetic activity of metoclopramide or dexamethasone. Am J Clin Oncol 1991 (14):238-242

6 Kris MG, Gralla RH, Tyson LB et al: Controlling delayed vomiting: double-blind randomised trial comparing placebo, dexamethasone alone and metoclopramide plus dexamethasone in patients receiving cisplatin. J Clin Oncol 1989 (7):108-114

7 Shinkai T, Saijo N, Eguchi K et al: Control of cisplatin-induced delayed emesis with metoclopramide and dexamethasone. A randomised trial. Jpn J Clin Oncol 1989 (19/1):40-44

8 Italian Group for Antiemetic Research: Cisplatin-induced delayed emesis: Pattern and prognostic factors during three subsequent cycles. Ann Oncol 1994 (5):585-589

9 Passalacqua R, Bella M, Monici L et al: Double-blind randomised trial for the control of delayed emesis: a comparison of placebo versus ACTH. Proc Am Soc Clin Oncol 1988 (9):1270

10 Jones AL, Hill AS, Soukop M et al: Comparison of dexamethasone and ondansetron in the prophylaxis of emesis induced by moderately emetogenic chemotherapy. Lancet 1991 (338):483-487

11 Kris MG, Tyson LB, Clark RA et al: Oral ondansetron for the control of delayed emesis after cisplatin. Cancer 1992 (70):1012-1016

12 De Mulder HM, Seynaeve C, Vermorken JB et al: Ondansetron compared with high-dose metoclopramide in prophylaxis of acute and delayed cisplatin-induced nausea and vomiting. Ann Int Med 1990 (113):834-840

13 Gandara DR: Progress in the control of acute and delayed emesis induced by cisplatin. Eur J Cancer 1991 (Suppl 1):S9-S11

14 Levitt M, Warr D, Yelle L et al: Ondansetron compared with dexamethasone and metoclopramide as antiemetics in the chemotherapy of breast cancer with cyclophosphamide, methotrexate and 5-fluorouracil. N Engl J Med 1993 (328):1081-1084

15 Kaizer L, Warr D, Hoskins P et al: The effect of schedule and maintenance on the antiemetic efficacy of ondansetron combined with dexamethasone in patients receiving moderately emetogenic chemotherapy. Proc Am Ass Clin Oncol 1992 (11):381

Prevention of Emesis from Radiotherapy

Terrence J. Priestman

The Radiotherapy Department, The Royal Hospital, Cleveland Road, Wolverhampton WV2 1BT, United Kingdom

Although the majority of patients undergoing radiotherapy as part of their cancer treatment will not experience sickness, there remains a substantial minority for whom nausea and vomiting will occur as distressing side-effects during their irradiation. For those patients who do develop problems, the degree of emesis varies considerably but is generally less severe than that associated with intensive chemotherapy. The duration of radiation-induced sickness may, however, be considerably longer than that associated with chemotherapy - since a course of radiotherapy may involve 30 to 40 fractions (treatments) over a period of 6 to 8 weeks and, if untreated, sickness could persist throughout this period. Thus whilst the emesis associated with therapeutic irradiation is not as severe or predictable as that seen with many cytotoxic drug regimens, the symptoms are still upsetting for the patient and require treatment.

Mechanisms of Radiation-Induced Emesis

The precise pathophysiology of radiation-induced emesis remains unclear. Animal models indicate that centrally two sites in the brain stem are involved: the area postrema and the vomiting centre. The area postrema is a highly vascular region, outside the blood-brain barrier, near the caudal floor of the fourth ventricle, which contains the chemoreceptor trigger zone and mediates the stimuli provided by emetic compounds carried in the blood or cerebrospinal fluid. These stimuli are then relayed to the nearby vomiting centre in the reticular formation of the medulla. The vomiting centre may also be stimulated directly by afferent fibres from the vagal nerve [1].

Destruction of the area postrema reduces sensitivity to radiation-induced emesis in dogs [2,3], inhibiting emesis at doses of 6 Gy to 8 Gy. At higher does of 15 Gy to 20 Gy, however, vomiting still occurs suggesting a role for the neuronal pathway. This would support older data showing that supradiaphragmatic vagotomy in monkeys significantly reduced radiation-induced vomiting [4] although similar studies in the dog showed little effect [5]. These results would seem to suggest that the area postrema is the most sensitive site for reception of emetic stimuli with visceral pathways having a secondary role [1].

Much work has been done to identify the neurotransmitters involved in the emetic reflex and the principal compounds involved include 5-hydroxytryptamine (5-HT), adrenaline, noradrenaline, dopamine, histamine and acetylcholine. It is now clear that there are a family of receptors for 5-HT and stimulation of different receptors will result in different responses. In 1978 it was shown that the 5-HT_3 receptor appeared to be involved in emesis when it was demonstrated that metoclopramide was a competitive antagonist of 5-HT, acting at this site [6]. Subsequent studies have confirmed the presence of high concentrations of 5-HT_3 receptors in both the chemoreceptor trigger zone [7] and vagal afferents [8]. Metoclopramide also inhibits dopamine receptors (which, clinically, may give rise to extrapyramidal toxicity) and so, following this observation, specific 5-HT_3 receptor antagonists were developed (such as ondansetron, tropisetron, dolasetron and granisetron) which have shown potent activity both in animal models and in the clinical situation, in inhibiting emesis (Fig.1).

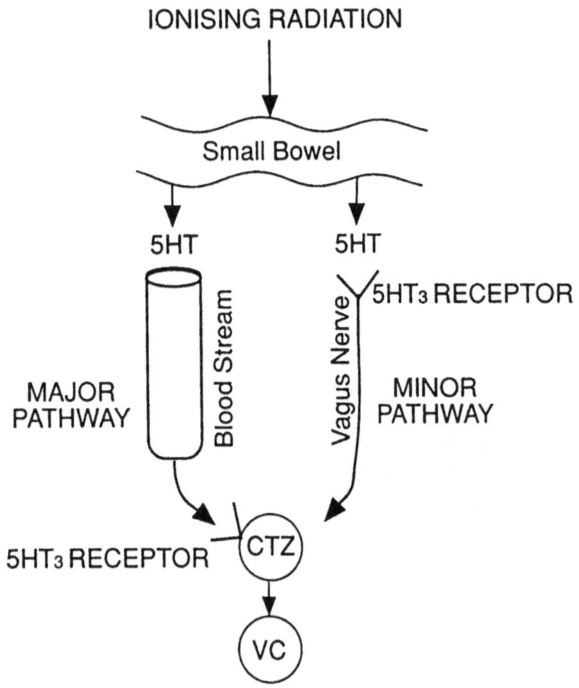

Fig. 1. Summary of postulated pathophysiology of radiation-induced emesis due to release of 5-hydroxytryptamine (5-HT)

Factors Predicting for Radiation-Induced Emesis

In purely practical terms a number of factors have been identified which help predict the likelihood of sickness developing during radiotherapy treatment. These include site, field size, dose per fraction, age, and level of anxiety.

Site

Patients having radiotherapy to the upper abdomen are most at risk of developing symptoms. Surprisingly, although this problem has been recognised since the earliest days of therapeutic irradiation, the actual incidence of emesis in this situation has never been accurately quantified, although in one series of patients undergoing hemi-body irradiation it was noted that following single doses of 8 Gy, with no antiemetic prophylaxis, 91% of those having upper-body irradiation and 33% receiving lower-body treatment experienced significant emesis [9]. Animal studies have confirmed that irradiation of the gut mucosa results in release of 5-HT from the enterochromaffin cells which may lead to direct stimulation of the chemoreceptor trigger zone or stimulation of vagal afferents resulting in emesis [10]. Despite these logical explanations it is still the case that a small but significant proportion of patients undergoing radiotherapy to other sites of the body, where such mechanisms cannot be invoked, do experience considerable emesis.

Field Size

In general terms the greater the volume of tissue being irradiated the greater the risk of sickness developing. The most obvious example of this is total-body irradiation for patients with leukaemias and lymphomas.

Dose per Fraction

The greater the dose given at each treatment the greater the risk of emesis. Most curative radiotherapy involves courses of daily treatment (5 days per week) for between 3 to 8 weeks with average daily doses of 1.8 to 3 Gy. Palliative radiation often comprises single-exposure treatments with doses of 8 to 15 Gy, greatly increasing the risk of emesis for these patients.

Age

It has been suggested that children are less susceptible to radiation-induced emesis than adults [11].

Anxiety

Although not well documented it has also been suggested that anxiety and apprehension may increase the likelihood of sickness in radiotherapy patients.

Despite the long-standing recognition of the problem of radiation-induced emesis there have been relatively few published studies regarding its control or prevention. This is in marked contrast to the now very extensive literature on chemotherapy-related sickness. A discussion of those trials which have been reported may be conveniently divided into two categories: series using established antiemetics and series using the new generation of antiemetics: the 5-HT_3 antagonists.

Studies with Established Antiemetics

In Britain at the present time metoclopramide is almost certainly the most widely used antiemetic for the control of radiation-induced emesis. Despite this pre-eminence there are only a handful of published studies on its efficacy in this indication other than recent comparative trials with 5-HT_3 antagonists; these latter results are considered later. In the former series an initial study looked at patients receiving upper abdominal radiotherapy during a fractionated course of treatment with daily doses of 2 Gy. All patients received metoclopramide 10 mg tds orally from the beginning of their treatment. Of the 30 patients evaluated, 14 had no nausea or vomiting throughout their course. Of the remainder 10 experienced minor emesis but did not require a change in therapy and 6 had symptoms controlled by metoclopramide for an average of 6 days but then developed more severe emesis and were given the cannabinoid nabilone as an alternative antiemetic; this controlled their sickness but gave rise to some toxicity [12].

This initial evaluation led to a randomised double-blind crossover study where patients who developed emesis during a fractionated course of radiotherapy were given either metoclopramide 10 mg tds orally or nabilone 1 mg bd (with a placebo tablet at mid-day). Fifty-two percent of those given nabilone felt they achieved good symptom control compared to 48% who received metoclopramide. A further 24% and 36%, respectively, felt that control was adequate and that they did not wish for any additional antiemetic therapy. These results obviously showed no significant difference in efficacy between the two drugs but nabilone caused significantly more toxicity than metoclopramide, which was well tolerated [13]. These results would suggest that appproximately 80% of patients who experience radiation-induced emesis will achieve good or adequate symptomatic relief with oral metoclopramide.

In a third study 89 patients who developed emesis during a course of radiotherapy were randomised to receive either metoclopramide 100 mg 4 hourly, prochlorperazine 10 mg 4 hourly, or a placebo. Surprisingly, assessments based on the number of vomits and a rating scale for nausea showed no significant differences between the 3 arms (although no precise figures for response were quoted). Less surpisingly, there was extensive toxicity with metoclopramide at this high dose, 21 of 28 (75%) patients experiencing side-effects, which were principally neurological [14].

Phenothiazine derivatives are also extensively employed, probably the most popular agent being prochlorperazine. Once again, however, apart from the series cited above and one other (small) study, the only published results with this drug in this indication come from randomised trials with 5-HT_3 antagonists. The former trial was a randomised cross-over comparison with the cannabinoid tetrahydrocannabinol in patients undergoing fractionated irradiation. Only 11 patients were randomised, however, and of these only 7 were evaluable: 4 of 7 noticed an improvement in symptoms with the cannabinoid and 3 with prochlorperazine [15].

Another, less frequently used phenothiazine, chlorpromazine, was evaluated in a randomised comparison with the cannabinoid levonantrodol [16]. In this series patients received either 25 mg of chlorpromazine or 0.5 or 0.75 mg of levonantrodol 30 minutes before single-exposure treatments of 10 to 15 Gy to the thoracic/lumbar spine or hypochondrium. Forty-three patients were entered, 7 of 14 (50%) in the chlorpromazine group vomited within 4 hours of irradiation compared with 17 of 29 (59%) given the cannabinoid. Although the numbers were small and no details on the severity of emesis were given, the authors' final conclusion that neither drug proved particularly effective was probably valid.

Cannabinoids enjoyed a brief vogue during the mid-1980s in the treatment of radiation-emesis and the 3 published studies assessing their efficacy are described above. Although nabilone appeared relatively active in this indication, its considerable toxicity resulted in its being abandoned in favour of less troublesome agents.

Domperidone is the only other agent to have received any attention in the literature in this situation. A review of unpublished data has reported on 7 patients given a course of abdominal irradiation, 17 who received thoracic radiotherapy and 6 who underwent total body irradiation. All patients had developed sickness during treatment and were given the drug at a dose of 10 to 20 mg tds. Only 14 (47%) had complete relief of symptoms and 6 (20%) had no benefit whatsoever [17].

Studies with 5-HT_3 Antagonists

These may be conveniently divided into trials based on conventional radiotherapy and those involving total body irradiation.

Trials with Conventional Radiotherapy

Two prospective double-blind randomised studies, both from Britain, have been reported comparing established antiemetics with a 5-HT_3 antagonist.

The more recent study looked at patients undergoing fractionated irradiation to the upper abdomen who were to receive 5 or more daily treatments with fraction sizes of 1.8 Gy or more. They were randomised to receive ondansetron 8 g tds or prochlorperazine 10 mg tds from 1 hour before their first treatment, as emesis prophylaxis. Assessment of emesis was by diary cards, completed by the patient, and responses in terms of emesis were graded as complete (no episodes of retching or vomiting), major (1-2 episodes), minor (3-5 episodes), or failure (more than 5 emetic episodes). Nausea was graded into 4 categories: none, mild, moderate or severe, based on the patients' own assessments.

There were 135 evaluable patients, 70 of whom received ondansetron and 65 prochlorperazine. As Table 1 shows, 61% of the patients on ondansetron had complete control of emesis throughout treatment compared to only 35% of those receiving the phenothiazine ($p<0.001$, 95% confidence limits 1.54, 5.07). The table also shows the number of emetic episodes patients experienced on their worst day during the study period and there were

Table 1. Odansetron versus prochlorperazine: number of emetic episodes on worst day during study

Number of emetic episodes	Ondansetron (n=70)	Prochlorperazine (n=65)
0	43 (61%)	2 (35%)
1	3 (4%)	13 (20%)
2	3 (4%)	6 (9%)
3	3 (4%)	3 (4%)
4	1 (1%)	1 (2%)
5	0	0
>5	17 (24%)	19 (29%)

Table 2. Odansetron versus prochlorperazine: degree of nausea on worst day during study

Nausea grade on worst day	Ondansetron (n=70)	Prochlorperazine (n=65)
None	23 (33%)	14 (22%)
Mild	16 (23%)	23 (35%)
Moderate	15 (21%)	9 (14%)
Severe	26 (23%)	19 (29%)

significantly fewer episodes in patients given ondansetron ($p=0.04$). However, almost a quarter of the ondansetron patients did experience more than 5 episodes of vomiting or retching on a single day and were thus treatment failures, indicating that prevention of troublesome emesis was far from complete in this group.

When nausea was considered there was no significant difference between the groups either for the grade of nausea experienced on the worst day during the study (Table 2) or the proportion of days during treatment when nausea was absent or mild, with about a quarter of the patients in both groups experiencing severe symptoms.

An earlier trial was based on single-exposure high-dose palliative treatments. Patients who were to receive single doses of 8 to 10 Gy to fields of at least 100 cm^2 of the upper abdomen (centred between T10 to L1) were randomised to receive either ondansetron 8 mg tds for 5 days or metoclopramide 10 mgs tds for a similar period. Both drugs were started 1 hour prior to

Table 3. Ondansetron verusus metoclopramide: Control of emesis in first 24 hours after single-exposure radiotherapy

Emetic control	**Complete**	**Major**	**Minor**	**Failure**
Ondansetron	45 (92%)	4 (8%)	0	0
Metoclopramide	26 (46%)	14 (25%)	7 (12%)	9 (16%)
Nausea	**None**	**Mild**	**Moderate**	**Severe**
Ondansetron	33 (67%)	10 (21%)	4 (8%)	1 (2%)
Metoclopramide	22 (39%)	12 (21%)	10 (18%)	12 (21%)

Table 4. Control of emesis during days 1 to 5 after single-exposure radiotherapy

Day	**1**	**2**	**3**	**4**	**5**
Ondansetron	100/88*	98/82	100/75	98/79	98/74
Metoclopramide	71/60	86/76	93/76	91/84	96/83

* all figures are percentages, the first relates to emetic control (complete or major), the second to nausea (none or mild)

irradiation and given orally. Assessment and grading of response was similar to that in the above study.

An interim analysis [19] was carried out after 97 patients had entered the trial, 84 of whom were evaluable. The results showed that in the first 24 hours after irradiation 97% of patients on ondansetron had complete control of emesis compared to only 46% of those given metoclopramide (p=0.001) during the same period. Seventy-three percent of those taking the 5-HT_3 antagonist had no nausea compared to only 41% taking metoclopramide (p=0.001). In view of these differences the trial was terminated at this point but during the period of the analysis randomisation had continued and a further 24 patients entered on study. A final analysis was therefore carried out to include these individuals [20]. Of the 121 subjects entered 105 were ultimately evaluable and the results are shown in Tables 3 and 4. As can be seen, the benefit of ondansetron remained highly significant, there was 100% either complete or major control of emesis on day 1, whereas 28% of those on metoclopramide failed to be controlled or achieved only minor control.

Days 2 to 5 were also analysed. Naturally over this period the emetic effect of the radiation was diminishing and the smaller differences between the two drugs did not reach statistical significance. However, emesis continued to be almost completely controlled by ondansetron, as shown in Table 4. Nausea, on the other hand, did persist in 10% to 20% of cases through days 2 to 5 and was not fully controlled by either drug.

In an open study, patients receiving fractionated upper-abdominal irradiation in daily doses of 1.8 to 4 Gy were given ondansetron, again at a dose 8 mg tds orally. Emesis was completely controlled in 19 of 20 patients throughout their radiation course [21].

A further non-randomised study assessed the value of a second 5-HT_3 anatagonist, granisetron, in the prevention of emesis when lower hemi-body irradiation was given. In this series, 22 patients with bone secondaries were given granisetron intravenously at a dose of either 20 µg/kg or 40 µg/kg 1 hour prior to a single midline dose of 8 Gy. A complete response (no nausea or vomiting) was noted in 9 of 13 (69%) patients at the lower dose level and 6 of 9 (66%) at the higher level [22]. The value of antiemetic therapy in this study is difficult to gauge as a previous series showed that only 33% of patients receiving single-dose, lower-half body irradiation would experience significant sickness [9].

Early results with tropisetron have also been reported in a series of 20 women receiving postoperative abdominal irradiation for ovarian cancer [23]. Twelve patients received radiotherapy to the whole abdomen (20 Gy in 4 weeks) plus a boost to the lower abdomen and pelvis (20 Gy in 2 weeks) and 8 received treatment to the lower abdomen and pelvis only (40 Gy in 5 weeks). Tropisetron was given throughout treatment at a dose of 5 mg daily. Vomiting was recorded on a weekly basis and the incidence ranged from 8% to 17% per week for those having whole-abdomen irradiation compared to 0 to 13% per week for the smaller field. The proportion of patients experiencing nausea each week ranged from 30% to 54% but overall quality of life was well maintained.

Studies in Total Body Irradiation (TBI)

Nausea and vomiting is almost universal after TBI and is equally prevalent whether treatment is given as a single dose or in a fractionated course with doses as low as 1.2 Gy daily, in spite of the use of conventional antiemetics such as metoclopramide [11,24]. Several non-randomised studies have made initial assessments of 5-HT_3 antagonists in this situation.

Two studies have used ondansetron and included both children and adults undergoing conditioning for bone marrow transplantation. The conditioning included both chemotherapy (with cyclophosphamide) and TBI, but separate assessments of emesis were made for the two components of the conditioning process. In the first study the radiation dose for children was 1.8 Gy twice daily for 4 days and they were given ondansetron 5 to 8 mg/m^2 iv during conditioning. For adults the regimen was 6 Gy for 2 doses or 8 Gy as a single dose with ondansetron 8 mg tds iv during conditioning. Among the children complete or major control of emesis was achieved in 9 of 11 (82%) during TBI whilst of the adults 74% had complete and 95% complete or major control [25]. In the second trial, confined to children below the age of 18, radiation was given at a dose of 6 Gy on 2 consecutive days immediately prior to transplantation, ondansetron was given at a dose of 8 mg tds iv. Here 59% and 81% of the patients had complete or major control of emesis during the first and second days of TBI, respectively, and complete or major control was maintained in 75% to 82% of patients thereafter [26].

A third study [27] evaluated granisetron in 32 consecutive patients receiving single fraction TBI at a dose of 7.5 Gy. Previous experience had indicated that 95% of such patients would suffer severe emesis despite the use of conventional antiemetics. All patients were aged 14 years or more and were given granisetron 40 µg/kg 30 to 60 minutes prior to irradiation with the option of 2 further doses over the next 24 hours if needed. Eighteen patients (56%) experienced total protection and a further 13 (41%) had major antiemetic protection. The criteria for the latter were, however, rather different from other studies cited here, but overall 70% of patients had no vomiting and nausea graded only as either none or mild. Only 3 patients required a second dose of granisetron.

Drug Safety

At the relatively low doses used for the relief of radiation-induced emesis, side-effects with metoclopramide and prochlorperazine are few and minor. Happily the new generation of 5-HT_3 antagonists appears to be equally well tolerated, no major toxicities have been reported, occasional headache and constipation are the only consistent adverse events to have been documented and these occur in less than 10% of patients in most series [19,22,27].

Conclusions

Recent clinical trials indicate that the 5-HT_3 receptor antagonist, ondansetron, has a clear superiority over agents such as prochlorperazine and metoclopramide in the prevention and control of radiation-induced emesis, with the abolition of vomiting and retching in more than 90% of patients at high risk of developing sickness after high-dose single-exposure treatments or TBI. Early indications are that the other 5-HT_3 antagonists will show similar levels of efficacy.

When given over longer periods, during fractionated radiotherapy, the results are less impressive with up to a quarter of patients still experiencing severe emesis and nausea control being no better than with conventional agents [18].

In chemotherapy studies the efficacy of 5-HT_3 antagonists has been enhanced by the addition of dexamethasone [27] and it is possible that the same might be true in radiotherapy. In a pilot study it has been shown that the combination of ondansetron and dexamethasone proved effective in preventing vomiting and nausea for patients undergoing hemi-body irradiation [28].

Ondansetron was the first 5-HT_3 antagonist to become commercially available in Britain and has now been joined by tropisetron and granisetron (although the latter is, as yet, only available in an intravenous formulation). Further similar drugs are under development. Future clinical trials with these agents are likely to be directed towards comparisons between the drugs and the assessment of combination antiemetic therapy with agents such as dexamethasone, in order to identify the optimum regimen for the prevention or relief of emesis caused by radiotherapy.

REFERENCES

1 Harding RK: Prodromal effects of radiation: pathways models and protection by antiemetics. Pharmac Ther 1988 (39):335-345

2 Harding RK, Hugenholtz H and Keaney M: Discrete lesions of the area postrema abolish radiation-induced emesis in the dog. Neurosci Lett 1985 (53):95-100

3 Harding RK: Prodromal effects of radiation: pathways, models and protection by antiemetics. Pharmac Therap 1988 (37):335-345

4 Brizzee KR: Effect of localized brain stem lesions and subdiaphragmatic vagotomy on x-irradiation emesis in the monkey. Am J Physiol 1956 (187):567-570

5 Carpenter DO, Briggs DB and Strominger NL: Radiation-induced emesis in the dog; effects of lesions and drugs. Radiat Res 1986 (108):307-316

6 Fozard JR and Mobarak Ali AT: Blockade of neuronal tryptaminase receptors by metoclopramide. Eur J Pharmacol 1978 (49):109-112

7 Higgins GA, Kilpatrick GJ, Buncwe KT, Jones BJ and Tyers M: B 5-HT3 receptor antagonists injected into the area postrema inhibit cisplatin induced emesis in the ferret. Br J Pharmacol 1989 (97):247-255

8 Richardson BP, Engel G, Donatsch P and Stadler PA: Identification of serotonin M-receptor subtypes and their specific blockade by a new class of drugs. Nature 1985 (316):126-131

9 Danjoux CE, Rider WD and Fitzpatrick PJ: The acute radiation syndrome - a memorial to William Michael Court-Brown. Clin Radiol 1979 (30):581-584

10 Gunning SJ, Gagan RM and Tyers MB: Cisplatin induces biochemical and histological changes in the small intestine of the ferret. Br J Pharmacol 1987 (90):135P

11 Westbrook C, Glaholm J and Barrett A: Vomiting associated with whole body irradation. Clin Radiol 1987 (38):263-266

12 Priestman T and Priestman S: An initial evaluation of nabilone in the control of radiotherapy-induced nausea and vomiting. Clin Radiol 1984 (35):265-266

13 Priestman S, Priestman T and Canney P: A double-blind randomised cross-over comparison of nabilone and metoclopramide in the control of radiation-induced nausea. Clin Radiol 1987 (38):543-544

14 Sokol GH, Greenberg HM, McCarthy S, Sledjeski L and Lyman G: Radiation induced nausea (RIN): the comparative efficacy of oral metoclopramide (M) versus prochlorperazine (P) and placebo. A double blind randomized study. Proc Amer Soc Clin Oncol 1986 (5):248 (abstract)

15 Ungerleider JT, Andrysiak TA, Fairbanks LA, Tesler AS and Parker RG: Tetrahydrocannabinol vs prochlorperazine. The effects of two antiemetics on patients undergoing radiotherapy. Radiology 1984 (150):598-599

16 Lucraft HH and Palmer MK: Randomised clinical trial of levonantradol and chlorpromazine in the prevention of radiotherapy induced vomiting. Clin Radiol 1982 (33):621-622

17 Reyntjens A: Domperidone as an anti-emetic: summary of research reports. Postgrad Med J 1979 (55 Suppl 1):50-54

18 Priestman TJ, Roberts JT and Upadhyaya BK: A prospective randomized double-blind trial comparing ondansetron versus prochlorperazine for the prevention of nausea and vomiting in patients undergoing fractionated radiotherapy. Clin Oncol 1993 (5):358-363

19 Priestman TJ, Roberts JT, Lucraft H, Collis CH, Adams M, Upadhyaya BK and Priestman S: Results of a randomized double blind comparative study of ondansetron and metoclopramide in the prevention of nausea and vomiting following high dose abdominal irradiation. Clin Oncol 1990 (2):71-75

20 Collis CH, Priestman TJ, Priestman S, Lucraft H, Roberts JT, Adams M and Upadhyaya BK: The final assessment of a randomized double blind comparative study of ondansetron vs metoclopramide in the prevention of nausea and vomiting following high dose upper abdominal irradiation. Clin Oncol 1991 (3):241-242

21 Franzen L, Israelsson G, Lomberg H, Modig H and Henriksson R: Ondansetron prevents emesis induced by fractionated radiotherapy. Eur J Cancer Clin Oncol 1991 (Suppl 2):S295 (abstract)

22 Logue JP, Magee B, Hunter RD and Murdoch RD: The antiemetic effect of granisetron in lower hemibody radiotherapy. Clin Oncol 1991 (3):247-249.

23 Sorbe B and Berglind A-M: Tropisetron, a new 5-HT3-receptor antagonist in the prevention of radiation-induced nausea, vomiting and diarrhoea. Drugs 1992 (43 Suppl 3):33-39

24 Spitzer TR, Deeg HJ, Torrisi J, Cottler-Fox M, Cahill R, Pickle L and Dubois A: Total body irradiation (TBI) induced emesis is universal after small-dose fractions (120cGy) and is not cumulative dose related. Proc Amer Soc Clin Oncol 1990 (9):50 (abstract)

25 Hewitt M, Croockewit S, Abram WP, Upadhyaya BK and Lane-Allman E: Ondansetron prophylaxis against emesis produced by total body irradiation and chemotherapy conditioning for bone marrow transplantation. Eur J Cancer Clin Oncol 1991 (Suppl 2):S294 (abstract)

26 Jurgens H, McQuade B: Ondansetron as prophylaxis for chemotherapy and radiotherapy induced emesis in children. Oncology 1992 (49): 279-285

27 Hunter AE, Prentice HG, Pothecary K, et al: Granisetron, a selective 5HT3 receptor antagonist, for the prevention of radiation induced emesis during total body irradiation. Bone Marrow Transplant 1991 (7):439-441

28 Smyth JF, Coleman RE and Nicolson M: Does dexamethasone enhance control of acute cisplatin induced emesis by ondansetron? BMJ 1991 (303): 1423-1426

29 Roberts JT and Priestman TJ: A review of ondansetron in the management of radiotherapy-induced emesis. Oncology 1993 (50):173-179

Antiemetic Therapy in Cancer Patients Submitted to Narcotic Analgesics

Fausto Roila [1], Enzo Ballatori [2] and Albano Del Favero [3]

1 Medical Oncology Division, Policlinico Monteluce, Via Brunamonti, 06122 Perugia
2 Medical Statistics Unit, Department of Internal Medicine and Public Health, University of L'Aquila
3 Institute of Internal Medicine and Oncological Sciences, Policlinico Monteluce, Via Brunamonti, 06122 Perugia, Italy

Clinical Relevance of the Problem

Nausea and vomiting are common and familiar side-effects of opioid drugs, but surprisingly few data on the incidence and characteristics of this phenomenon in cancer patients can be found in the literature. In the few studies available the percentage of patients suffering opioid-related emesis varied from 2.7% [1] to 40% [2].

An Italian study that evaluated for 3 consecutive days 260 cancer patients receiving different orally administered narcotic analgesics (buprenorphine, morphine, codeine, oxycodone) but not receiving prophylactic antiemetic treatment provides useful information [3]. Patients with no emesis or nausea prior to narcotic therapy who experienced moderate or severe nausea and/or two or more emetic episodes during the 72 hours following the start of narcotic therapy were considered to have narcotic-induced gastrointestinal side-effects. Nausea/vomiting was reported by 8.3%/22.7% of patients treated with buprenorphine, by 18.3%/28% of those treated with morphine, by 16.2%/29.7% treated with codeine and by 10.0%/40.0% treated with oxycodone. Overall, 12.3% of patients had nausea and 26.5% had emesis; 22% had to interrupt the opioid analgesic. A different emetic incidence among the various narcotic analgesics was not demonstrated, but this problem can be resolved only by studying a very large patient population.

In another study 21.6% of patients treated with oral morphine and all receiving prophylactic antiemetics (e.g. prochlorperazine) suffered emesis [4].

All clinically useful μ-agonist opioids produce some degree of nausea and vomiting. Careful, controlled clinical studies comparing the efficacy and tolerability of opioids have demonstrated that in equianalgesic dosages the incidence of such side-effects was not significantly lower than that seen with morphine [5].

Certain individuals never vomit after morphine whereas others do so each time the drug is administered, but data on patient- or treatment-related factors able to explain these differences are at best scanty. Sex, patient's physical status and route of administration of opioids can be prognostic factors for opioid-induced emesis.

In fact, emesis is more frequent in females than males [4]; it is uncommon in recumbent patients while nausea is present in 40% and vomiting in 15% of ambulatory patients [5]. The route of administration may also be important. Patients receiving intramuscular morphine have emesis more frequently than after intravenous administration. Contrasting data are available on the emetogenic effects of epidural and intrathecal administration of opioids. While in some studies this modality of administration was found to be associated with a high incidence of emetic symptoms [6], in others these side-effects were not particularly troublesome [7].

Pathogenesis

Since many years it has been recognised that opioid drugs can provoke nausea and vomiting. Nevertheless, the exact pathogenic mechanism of opioid-induced emesis is still unclear and its identification is further complicated by the fact that opioids can exert both emetic and antiemetic action. However, the awareness that multiple opioid receptors exist and that many neurotransmitters can be involved in opioid-induced emesis helped to clarify, at least in part, this rather confusing matter.

Experimental evidence suggests that the emetic effect of opioids is due to stimulation of the receptors within the medullary chemoreceptor trigger zone; in fact, its ablation prevented vomiting in animals [2], but a peripheral mechanism due to constipation and delayed gastric emptying may also be involved. Instead, the antiemetic effect is probably related to an action on μ and/or κ receptors [8].

Many neurotransmitters are considered to be involved in opioid-induced emesis: dopamine, histamine and perhaps serotonin. Dopamine release from dopaminergic nerves in several brain areas can be induced by morphine acting via receptors [9]. Intraventricular pretreatment with the opioid antagonist naloxone, histamine H1 and H2 antagonists gave protection from emesis induced by intracerebroventricularly administered morphine. Furthermore, the CSF histamine concentration was significantly raised 5 min after morphine administration [10]. The role of serotonin is still uncertain. Although in man a possible involvement of the 5-HT_3 receptors has been suggested [11], in the ferret one study showed that emesis induced by morphine and morphine-6-glucuronide was not abolished or reduced by some 5-HT_3 antagonists [12], while in another study it was significantly decreased with high-dose ondansetron but not granisetron [13]. Although the ferret is thought to be a good model for emesis induced by cytotoxic drugs and radiation in man, this might not be the case for opioid-like compounds. Whether there is interaction between the neurotransmitters and whether one of these has a peculiar role is still unknown.

The emetic action of opioids is further complicated by the above mentioned antiemetic effect which is probably mediated via a medullary antiemetic centre [14,15]. An antiemetic effect of low-dose morphine has been shown in the cat [14], while in the dog high-dose morphine fails to induce emesis and acts as an antiemetic against cytotoxic-induced emesis [12].

Another unsolved problem is whether the opioid drug or its metabolite is responsible for the emetic effect. In the ferret morphine 6-glucuronide, a metabolite of morphine, showed greater emetic potency than morphine [12], but this does not seem the case in man [16]; furthermore, no relationship between plasma levels of morphine and morphine 6-glucuronide and emetic response has been shown in the ferret [12].

Antiemetic Therapy

Despite the extensive use of opioid drugs in cancer patients appropriate studies on the use of antiemetic drugs to control opioid-induced emesis are at best scanty, Therefore, the use of antiemetic drugs is based more on personal experience than on scientific evidence.

Some authors always combine one (or more) antiemetic with opioids [4], while others do not prescribe an antiemetic in anticipation of opioid-induced emesis [17]. In fact, in one study more than 25% of patients required 2 or 3 antiemetic drugs [4] while in another study 29% of patients did not require an antiemetic and fewer than 10% required more than one antiemetic [17]. Furthermore, although it is common experience that nausea and emesis are initiation side-effects of opioids that resolve with continued use (tolerance), no studies have evaluated if antiemetic treatment could be interrupted or if it was necessary to continue for the full duration of opioid treatment.

In general, use of drug therapy is more successful for prophylaxis of vomiting than for treatment. Oral dosage forms are most useful for prophylaxis; suppository and parenteral forms are preferred for treatment. Haloperidol, metoclopramide, H1 antagonists and prochlorperazine are the most commonly used antiemetic drugs, but no comparative data are yet available. Haloperidol (1-2 mg orally every 12 hours) is sometimes preferred because, due to its longer half-life, it requires fewer administrations and induces less sedation than prochlorperazine (5 mg orally every 4-8 hours). On the other hand, metoclopramide (10 mg orally every 4 hours) is preferred when enhanced gastric emptying and a non-sedative effect is desired.

H1 antagonists with prominent anticholinergic properties (diphenhydramine) may be particularly useful in ambulatory patients or in addition to neuroleptics to counteract the extrapyramidal side-effects of the latter.

Experience with the new 5-HT_3 antagonists is still very limited. As mentioned before, an interesting pilot study using ondansetron has recently been published. In patients submitted to opioids and with emesis refractory to common antiemetics (metoclopramide, alizapride, domperidone plus dexamethasone) 5 out of 6 obtained complete control of vomiting with 16-32 mg/day orally administered ondansetron [11].

Conclusions

More epidemiological studies are needed to better define the incidence, intensity, starting time and duration of opioid-induced emesis. To identify the best treatment, prospective double-blind trials comparing antiemetic drugs vs placebo are needed. However, despite all these limits, some practical guidelines can be provided.

Firstly, in our opinion the apparently low incidence of opioid-induced emesis does not justify the routine prophylactic use of antiemetics. Secondly, if prophylactic treatment is needed, the possible tolerance to the emetic effect of opioids should be considered. Thirdly, if nausea and vomiting occur after the start of opioid analgesics, one of the old emetic drugs alone or in combination can be used. The choice should be based on their different pharmacokinetic and side-effect profiles. Finally, due to its high cost, the use of ondansetron is justifiable only in patients with nausea or vomiting not responsive to one or more of the old antiemetic drugs.

REFERENCES

1 Spector R: Analgesia. In: Spector R (ed) The Scientific Basis of Clinical Pharmacology. Little Brown, Boston 1986 pp 343-354

2 Mitchelson F: Pharmacological agents affecting emesis. A review (part I). Drugs 1992 (43):295-315

3 Campora E, Merlini L, Pace M, Bruzzone M, Luzzani M, Gottlieb A, Rosso R: The incidence of narcotic-induced emesis. J Pain Symptom Management 1991 (6):428-430

4 Walsh TD: Antiemetic drug combinations in advanced cancer. Lancet 1982 (i):1018

5 Jaffe JH and Martin WR: Opioid analgesics and antagonists. In: Goodman Gillman A et al (eds) The Pharmacological Basis of Therapeutics. 8th Ed. Pergamon Press, New York 1990 pp 485-521

6 Cousins MJ, Mather LE: Intrathecal and epidural administration of opioids. Anesthesiology 1984 (61): 276-310

7 Zenz M, Piepenbrock S, Tryba M: Epidural opiates: long-term experiences in cancer pain. Klin Wochenschr 1985 (63):225-229

8 Blancquaert JP, Lefebvre RA, Willems JL: Emetic and antiemetic effects of opioids in the dog. Eur J Pharmacol 1986 (128):143-150

9 Chesselet MF, Chéramy A, Reisine TD, Glowinsky J: Morphine and δ-opiate agonists locally stimulate in vivo dopamine release in the cat caudate nucleus. Nature 1981 (291):320-322

10 Gupta YK, Bhandari P, Chugh A, Seth SD, Dixit KS, Bhargava KP: Role of endogenous opioids and histamine in morphine induced emesis. Indian J Exp Biol 1989 (27):52-54

11 Gottlieb A and Luzzani M: Il problema della nausea e del vomito da oppiacei nel paziente neoplastico avanzato: nuovo approccio farmacologico con gli antagonisti dei recettori 5-HT3. Studio preliminare. In: Proceedings of the International Congress "Il trattamento della nausea e del vomito da chemioterapia antineoplastica: nuove acquisizioni sul ruolo dei 5-HT3 antagonisti". Verona, 18 June 1991, pp 127-131

12 Thompson PI, Bingham S, Andrews PLR, Patel N, Joel SP, Slevin ML: Morphine 6-glucuronide: a metabolite of morphine with greater emetic potency than morphine in the ferret. Br J Pharmacol 1992 (106): 3-10

13 Wynn RL, Essien E, Thut PD: The effects of different antiemetic agents on morphine-induced emesis in ferrets. Eur J Pharmacol 1993 (241):47-54

14 Costello DJ and Borison HL: Naloxone antagonizes narcotic self-blockade of emesis in the cat. J Pharmacol Exp Ther 1977 (203):222-230

15 Harris AL: Cytotoxic-therapy-induced vomiting is mediated via enkephalin pathways. Lancet 1982 (i): 714-716

16 Osborne RJ, Slevin MI, Joel SP, Trew DM, Thompson PI, Malpas JS: The analgesic activity and pharmacokinetics of morphine and morphine-6-glucuronide in man. Br J Cancer 1989 (60): 451

17 Hanks GW: Antiemetics for terminal cancer patients. Lancet 1982 (i):1410

Antiemetic Therapy in Paediatric Patients

Richard F. Stevens

Royal Manchester Children's Hospital, Pendlebury, Manchester M27 4HA, United Kingdom

The past three decades have been associated with a dramatic increase in the cure rate for children with malignant disease. This improvement has been the result of, in the main, more intensive chemotherapy and radiotherapy regimens which have been associated with increased toxicity, in particular acute side-effects due to myelosuppression, alopecia and nausea and vomiting.

Implications of Chemotherapy-Related Nausea and Vomiting

Nausea and vomiting associated with chemotherapy can be severe and continue for several days after treatment has stopped [1]. This can lead to dehydration and electrolyte imbalance which has the potential for increasing the nephrotoxicity of chemotherapeutic agents such as cisplatinum [2].
In cancer patients, nausea (the sensation of the imminent need to vomit) and vomiting itself (for forceful expulsion of gastric contents) are not the mild, transient symptoms associated with other disease states. Rather, they may be severe and prolonged. These symptoms may become debilitating and children may become physically incapable of receiving further cancer chemotherapy or become so distressed physically and psychologically that they or their parents may consider refusal of further treatment. Many patients consider nausea and vomiting as the most distressing side-effects of cancer treatment (Table 1). It has been estimated that these symptoms can result in 25% to 50% of adult patients delaying one or more scheduled courses of chemotherapy or even refusing their treatment [4].

Factors Affecting Chemotherapy and Radiotherapy-Induced Emesis

Although not every patient receiving chemotherapy will experience nausea and vomiting, it has been estimated that this may occur in up to 70% of patients [5]. It is also well recognised that children are more prone to vomiting than adults [6].
By far the most important factor relating to drug-induced emesis is the nature of the chemotherapy received. Table 2 gives an indication of the emetogenic potential of chemotherapeutic drugs. These can range from the high-dose platinum drugs which cause emesis in the vast majority of children to weak emetogens such as the vinca alkaloids. It is not surprising that the dose, schedule and route of administration of these cytotoxics can also influence their emetogenic potential. Combination chemotherapy given over several days tends to have the greatest effect.

Table 1. Rank order of the side-effects of chemotherapy

Vomiting
Nausea
Alopecia
Thought of impending treatment
Timetable for treatment in clinic
Need for a needle
Breathlessness
Feeling tired
Difficulty with sleeping
etc.

data from Coates et al. [3]

Table 2. The emetogenic potential of commonly used chemotherapy and radiotherapy in children

HIGH POTENTIAL		Carboplatin
		Cisplatin
	A	High-dose cyclophosphamide (> 1 g/m^2)
		High-dose cytosine arabinoside
		Ifosfamide
		Total body irradiation
		Actinomycin D
		Adriamycin
		Busulphan
		Cyclophosphamide (0.5 to 1 g/m^2)
		Cytosine arabinoside (100 to 500 mg/m^2)
	B	Daunorubicin
		Epirubicin
		M-AMSA
		High-dose methotrexate (> 3 g/m^2)
		Mitoxantrone
		Procarbazine
		Low-dose cyclophosphamide (< 0.5 g/m^2)
		Low-dose cytosine arabinoside (< 100 mg/m^2)
	C	Methotrexate (< 3 g/m^2)
		Intrathecal triple chemotherapy
		Chest, abdominal, spinal radiotherapy
		L-asparaginase
		Bleomycin
	D	Vinblastine
		Vincristine
LOW POTENTIAL		VP 16 (etoposide)

Other factors can contribute towards emesis. Whether a child is new to chemotherapy or has received treatment before can affect their susceptibility to nausea and vomiting. Poor control of emesis during previous chemotherapy increases the incidence of nausea and vomiting during subsequent courses [7]. Bad experiences of emesis [8], anxiety [9] and a susceptibility to motion sickness [10] can also contribute towards emesis. Anticipatory vomiting is sometimes a problem and is usually the result of conditioning and may occur before the administration of subsequent courses of chemotherapy [11].

The pattern of emesis is not the same for all cytotoxic agents or modes of radiotherapy. Acute post-chemotherapy emesis has been most extensively studied and occurs during the first 24 hours after administration of the cytotoxic agent. It usually results in the most severe emesis and may well be associated with nausea and vomiting which starts the day after treatment and continues for several days (delayed emesis) [12]. The pattern of acute emesis can depend on the type of chemotherapy. For example, cisplatin tends to cause a peak of emesis 4 to 8 hours post-therapy, while high-dose cyclophosphamide and carboplatin cause peaks of emesis 10 to 12 hours post-treatment [13].

Emesis associated with radiotherapy is usually associated with irradiation of the epigastric region or upper abdomen or is associated with total body irradiation (TBI). The level of emesis tends to be dose related and adults tend to be more susceptible than children [14].

Clinical Presentation

Emesis associated with cytotoxic chemotherapy and radiotherapy can be very variable both in the symptoms that present and their intensity. These variations are the result of differences in patients' responses to identical regimens as well as the wide variety of treatment regimens involved. It is important therefore to evaluate the emetogenic potential of the therapy being used before initiating antiemetic therapy (see Table 2).

Symptoms range from nausea to retching and vomiting and frequently occur in a cyclic fashion if not treated early and effectively. Retching is the result of the same physiological mechanisms as vomiting, but there is no expulsion of gastric contents. Children often find retching more distressing than vomiting because of strain on the abdominal muscles and no apparent relief of symptoms.

The cyclical nature of nausea and vomiting is particularly important in the context of psychogenic or anticipation symptoms. Anticipatory emesis may occur at any time before treatment starts and is frequently very difficult to treat because it is usually the result of a conditioned response. It is therefore important to try and control emesis during the early courses of therapy.

Therapeutic Principles

There are three main aspects to the cytotoxic emesis in children: prophylaxis, duration of therapy, and individualisation of treatment.

Prophylaxis

The aim of prophylactic therapy is to block the receptor site before stimulation by the emetogenic agent and therefore treatment must be started prior to chemotherapy or radiotherapy. All antiemetics are more effective when used prophylactically, but the exact time for starting therapy depends on the type of chemotherapy, the patient's previous pattern of emesis and the route of administration of the antiemetic. Better and more rapid control can be achieved when antiemetics are given parenterally and the intravenous route is most commonly used as patients are often thrombocytopenic and frequently require venous access for the subsequent chemotherapy. Oral therapy has obvious advantages to patients and staff but may not be as effective in achieving emesis control.

Duration of Therapy

Once control of emesis has been achieved (often the result of achieving effective blood levels), it is important to maintain control by adopting a regular rather than an on-demand (PRN) approach. "Breakthrough" vomiting can be particularly difficult to treat. When parenteral therapy is indicated, a loading dose followed by regular therapy is the most appropriate, regardless of the patient's symptoms. The duration of therapy is dependent on the patient's previous pattern of emesis and the expected duration of the emesis based on the nature and dose of chemo-radiotherapy.

Individualisation of Treatment

Not all antiemetic regimens are effective in all patients. Table 2 lists some of the antineoplastic drugs used in the treatment of childhood malignancy in decreasing order of their emetogenic potential. The chemotherapeutic agents at the lower end of the scale may induce moderate nausea with little or no associated vomiting whereas those at the upper end may produce debilitating nausea accompanied by severe vomiting.

The severity of vomiting also differs between patients, with some patients experiencing a moderate number of emetic episodes over several days whereas others may show a very large number of episodes over just a few hours. Symptoms may appear almost instantaneously after chemotherapy or may be delayed for several hours. Combination chemotherapy increases the potential for more severe and prolonged emesis.

The psychological status of the patient also has an important role in formulating therapy. Positive suggestion (e.g. close proximity to another vomiting child) and the placebo effect of therapy are well recognised [15]. Children who suffer particularly from motion sickness are more prone to the side-effects of cancer chemotherapy [16]. Hypnosis or desensitisation may also be helpful additions in the control of emesis [17]. Conditioned patient responses, such as vomiting soon after arrival at the clinic, are difficult to control, but a friendly atmosphere that offers calm, privacy and reassurance to the patient without obvious stimuli such as the sight or smell of food, help considerably.

Table 3. Drugs used in the management of childhood emesis associated with chemo-radiotherapy

Class	Example	Mode of Action	Side-Effects
Phenothiazines	Chlorpromazine Prochlorperazine	Dopamine blockade at chemoreceptor trigger zone (CTZ), plus variable cholinergic and adrenergic receptor blockade	Extrapyramidal reactions, sedation, dry mouth
Antihistamines	Promethazine Cyclizine	Exact mode of action unknown. Block labyrinthine impulses. Sedative effect	Drowsiness
Dopamine	Metoclopramide Domperidone	Dopamine receptor blockade at CTZ. Increase in gastric emptying	Extrapyramidal reactions, sedation, diarrhoea
Butyrophenones	Haloperidol Droperidol	Dopamine receptor blockage at CTZ	Extrapyramidal reactions, sedation
Cannabinoids	Nabilone	Central antiemetic action - site unknown	Hypotension, dizziness, CNS disturbance
Corticosteroids	Methylprednisolone Dexamethasone	Uncertain, reduced prostaglandin synthesis	Dyspepsia, fluid retention
Benzodiazepines	Lorazepam	Central antiemetic action - site unknown	Sedation, respiratory depression
5-HT3 receptor antagonists	Ondansetron Granisetron	Blocking of selective 5-HT3 receptor sites both centrally and in the GI tract	Few and mild. Some constipation and headaches

The Pharmacological Approach to the Control of Emesis

As already mentioned, until recently there has been a relatively poor understanding of the basis of chemotherapy-induced emesis; antiemetics were frequently prescribed empirically. Which drug to use was based mainly on overt symptoms rather than on an accurate knowledge of the underlying physiology. For example, sedation and a reduced level of anxiety were found to relieve symptoms and therefore various benzodiazepines have been used. Dopamine antagonists which stimulate gastric motility have been shown to be effective in relieving the nausea associated with gastric stasis. Steroids are known to produce a "feeling of well-being" and may help control emesis.

Table 3 illustrates some of the diverse range of compounds which have been used as antiemetics. This list is not comprehensive and is influenced by availability and marketing in different parts of the world. Some of the drugs also go under different non-generic names.

Phenothiazines

Until recently the phenothiazines were the most widely used antiemetics in children. They exert dopamine blockade at the chemoreceptor trigger zone (CTZ) and may also directly depress the vomiting centre. They also exert variable cholinergic and adrenergic receptor blockade. Chlorpromazine is the best example of the aliphatic class. It has limited antiemetic activity and has a relatively high incidence of side-effects including hypotension, sedation, liver abnormalities, blood dyscrasias and unwanted potentiation of the sedative effects of narcotics and barbiturates. The piperazine class includes prochlorperazine, perphenazine, trifluoperazine and thiethylperazine. These agents have greater antiemetic action and produce less sedation. However, side-effects are common in children and result mainly from dopamine antagonism and are manifest clinically by a variety of extrapyramidal reactions including restlessness, akathisia (involuntary limb shaking), torticollis and oculogyric crises [18]. These reactions may be controlled by drugs such as diphenhydramine or lorazepam, but this is obviously undesirable.

Antihistamines

Although many antihistamines have antiemetic potential there is no real correlation between antiemetic activity and antihistamines. Promethazine and cyclizine are worth consideration in the control of mild to moderate emesis, particularly in the younger child and where a sedative effect would be useful.

Metoclopramide

Metoclopramide is a derivative of procamamide. It has central action by blocking dopamine receptors at the CTZ and also increases gastric emptying. It has a spectrum of activity resembling that of the phenothiazines, but its additional effect on the gut offers advantages. In adults undergoing chemo-radiotherapy there has been a tendency to increase the dose of metoclopramide with the aim of achieving better control of emesis. This has resulted in a higher incidence of side-effects, particularly extrapyramidal reactions [19], and has not proved a popular approach in children.

Domperidone

Domperidone also acts at the CTZ. It has no effect on gastric emptying but has the advantage over metoclopramide and the phenothiazines of being less likely to cause central effects such as sedation or dystonic reactions because it does not readily cross the blood-brain barrier.

Butyrophenones

Droperidol is a potent blocker of dopamine receptors at the CTZ. Experience of its use in children is limited. When used in higher doses it does have some antiemetic activity, but side-effects including tachycardia, agitation, somnolence and in particular extrapyramidal reactions are not uncommon. Haloperidol is also sometimes used as an antiemetic but it is not recommended for children.

Cannabinoids

The cannabinoids, the active ingredients of marijuana, have proven antiemetic properties. Although the exact mechanism of action is unknown, it is thought that they exert their effect via CNS depression. Nabilone is a synthetic cannabinoid and may be particularly useful in older children but side-effects including drowsiness, dizziness and the development of a "high" are not uncommon [20].

Corticosteroids

The exact mode of action of corticosteroids is unknown although it is suggested that stabilisation of lyposomal membranes may reduce prostaglandin synthesis. Dexamethasone has been most widely studied and appears to be most effective when used in combination [21, 22]. It appears to be a safe, effective adjunct to antiemetic regimens and should be evaluated further.

Benzodiazepines

Lorazepam has little or no direct antiemetic activity. However, it is sometimes useful when used in combination as it produces retrograde amnesia and can reduce anticipatory nausea and vomiting by reducing patients' previous experiences with chemotherapy [23].

5-HT$_3$ Antagonists

The mode of action of these new agents has already been discussed. In summary, they probably prevent emesis by blocking 5-HT$_3$ receptors at two sites: 1) the vagal afferent nerves that innervate the gastrointestinal tract, and 2) the same vagal nerves in the chemoreceptor trigger zone (CTZ) and hindbrain vomiting system.

At the present time only two 5-HT_3 antagonists are available, ondansetron (which is available in both oral and intravenous formulations) and granisetron (which is only available intravenously). Granisetron does not yet have a product licence for use in children and therefore the paediatric experience with the 5-HT_3 antagonists is based predominantly on ondansetron.

Ondansetron has been used in comparative and non-comparative studies [24]. Analysis of efficacy is complicated by the variety and complicity of chemotherapy but overall at least two-thirds of patients experience less than 3 emetic episodes on their "worst day" of chemotherapy (which can last up to 10 days) with cisplatin, ifosfamide and cyclophosphamide and total body irradiation. At least 80% of children experienced better control with ondansetron than previously with alternative antiemetics.

In many patients, good antiemetic control can be established with intravenous therapy and the continuing control maintained with oral medication [25]. There is also the potential for dose modification and other combinations (e.g. 5-HT_3 antagonists and dexamethasone) in particularly difficult patient groups.

The 5-HT_3 antagonists appear to be very well tolerated and lacking in major side-effects. Mild headaches, constipation and transient alterations in liver function tests have been reported [24], but extrapyramidal reactions appear absent. These agents have significant cost implications and therefore many oncology units are formulating their own criteria for their use. However, they have helped significantly in the control of emesis and influenced the overall quality of life for children undergoing intensive chemotherapy [26].

Table 4. Outline of emesis control in children

Emetogenic potential (on scale A to D, see Table 2 for details)	**Younger children**	**Older children**
High **A**	**Before therapy** 5-HT3 antagonist i.v. with or without dexamethasone i.v.	**Before therapy** 5-HT3 antagonist i.v. with or without dexamethasone i.v.
	After therapy 5-HT3 antagonist i.v. or oral +/- dexamethasone +/- metoclopramide	**After therapy** 5-HT3 antagonist i.v. or oral +/- dexamethasone +/- prochlorperazine
B	**Before therapy** 5-HT3 antagonist i.v.	**Before therapy** 5-HT3 antagonist i.v.
	After therapy 5-HT3 antagonist i.v. or oral +/- metoclopramide	**After therapy** 5-HT3 antagonist i.v. or oral +/- metoclopramide
C	Metoclopramide oral or i.v.	Prochlorperazine oral or i.v. or promethazine i.v.
D	No medication	No medication

Notes:
1) consider moving upwards to the next level if recent antiemetic failure;
2) consider moving sideways if borderline age;
3) consider use of lorazepam if anticipatory nausea and vomiting;
4) consider use of 5-HT3 antagonists on days of most emetogenic therapy;
5) do not use dexamethasone a) if chemotherapy includes steroids, or b) for brain tumours

Approach to Therapy

Every paediatric oncology unit should formulate its own policy for the control of emesis. There will be centre differences dependent on many factors including ward environment, nursing and psychological support, patient diagnostic profile, etc.
Table 4 outlines a possible approach to emesis control based on Table 2 where drugs are graded from highly emetogenic (group A) down to mildly emetogenic (group D). This table should only be considered as an outline but it does offer a basic structure which can be modified on the basis of local circumstances and newer developments.

Future Approaches

Problems in the control of emesis in children remain. Nausea and vomiting associated with the highly emetogenic drugs are still difficult to control. Different drug dosing and combinations are required. Alternative and complementary therapies such as hypnosis, relaxation therapy and acupuncture should be considered. Some of these modalities could be provided by parents, relatives and even siblings with the aim of achieving a more relaxed patient environment. Unfortunately these alternatives are often very time consuming.
It is hoped that the recent progress in the understanding of the physiology of emesis will continue and therefore provide a more scientific and rational background to the development of further antiemetic agents.

Conclusions

There is no one antiemetic agent or regimen currently available that will totally prevent chemotherapy-induced emesis in all patients. However, careful attention to the individual needs of the child and a knowledge of the previous pattern of nausea and vomiting followed by implementation of prophylactic and continuous therapy and a willingness to evaluate the newer and more physiological agents will increase the effectiveness of any antiemetic regimen.
For many years emesis has been one of the Cinderellas of medical oncology and has been judged with a higher priority by patients than possibly their health-care workers. A better understanding of the underlying physiology of emesis has enabled a more rational approach with more effective agents which have fewer side-effects. This has resulted in considerable improvement in the quality of life for many patients.

REFERENCES

1 Kris MG, Gralla RJ, Clark RA et al: Incidence, course and severity of delayed nausea and vomiting following the administration of high-dose cisplatin. J Clin Oncol 1985 (3):1379-1384

2 Madias NE and Harrington JT: Platinum nephrotoxicity. Am J Med 1978 (65):307-314

3 Coates A, Abraham S, Kaye SB et al: On the receiving end - patient perception of the side-effects of cancer chemotherapy. Eur J Cancer Oncol 1983 (19):203-208

4 Laszlo J: Nausea and vomiting as major complications of cancer chemotherapy. Drugs 1983 (25 Suppl 1):1-7

5 Morrow GR: Chemotherapy related nausea and vomiting: etiology and management. CAA Cancer Treat J 1989 (39):89-104

6 Roila F, Tonato M, Basurto C: Antiemetic activity of high doses of metochlopramide in cisplatin treated cancer patients: a randomised double-blind trial of the Italian Oncology Group for Clinical Research. J Clin Oncol 1988 (5):141-149

7 Marty M: Ondansetron and chemotherapy-induced emesis. 3rd National Congress on Neo-adjustment Chemotherapy. Paris, 1991

8 Andrykowsky MA, Redd WH, Hatfield AK: Development of anticipatory nausea: a prospective analysis. J Consult Clin Psychol 1985 (53):447-454

9 Nesse RM, Carli T, Curtis GC et al: Pre-treatment nausea in cancer chemotherapy: a conditioned response? Psychosom Med 1990 (42):43-46

10 Morrow GR: The assessment of nausea and vomiting. Cancer 1984 (53 Suppl 1):2267-2280

11 Morrow GR and Morrell CM: Behavioural treatment for the anticipatory nausea and vomiting induced by cancer chemotherapy. N Engl J Med 1982 (307): 1476-1480

12 Kris MG, Gralla RJ, Clark RA et al: Incidence, course and severity of delayed nausea and vomiting following the administration of high-dose cisplatin. J Clin Oncol 1985 (3):1379-1384

13 Martin M, Diaz-Rubio E, Sanches A et al: The natural course of emesis after carboplatin treatment. Acta Oncol 1990 (29S):593-595

14 Priestman T: Radiation-induced emesis. Clinician 1988 (6/3):40-43

15 Parson JA, Webster JH, Dowd J: Evaluation of the placebo effect in the treatment of radiation sickness. Acta Radiol 1961 (56):129-140

16 Morrow GR: The effect of a susceptibility to motion sickness on the side effects of cancer chemotherapy. Cancer 1985 (55):2766-2770

17 Zelter L, Le Baron S, Zelter PM: The effectiveness of behavioural intervention for reduction of nausea and vomiting in children and adolescents receiving chemotherapy. J Clin Oncol 1984 (2):683-690

18 Silva KL, Muller PJ, Pearce J: Acute drug-induced extrapyramidal syndromes. Practitioner 1973 (211):316-320

19 Gralla RJ, Itri LM, Pisko SE et al: Anti-emetic efficacy of high dose metaclopramide: randomised trials with placebo and prochlorperazine in patients with chemotherapy induced nausea and vomiting. N Engl J Med 1981 (305):905-909

20 Sallan SE, Cronin CM, Zelen M et al: Antiemetics in patients receiving chemotherapy for cancer. N Engl J Med 1989 (302):134-138

21 Bruera ED, Roca E, Cedara L et al: Improved control of chemotherapy induced emesis by addition of dexamethasone to metoclopramide in patients resistant to metoclopramide. Cancer Treat Rep 1983 (67):381

22 Drapkin RL, Sokol GH, Paladine WJ et al: The anti-emetic effect and dose response of dexamethasone in patients receiving cisplatinum. Proc Am Soc Clin Oncol 1982 (199):61

23 Laszlo J, Clark RA, Hanson DC: Lorazepam in cancer patients treated with cisplatin: A drug having antiemetic, amnesic and anxiolytic effects. J Clin Oncol 1985 (3):864-869

24 Stevens RF: A review of ondansetron as prophylaxis for chemotherapy and radiotherapy induced emesis in children. In: "Ondansetron" - Clinical Experience in Adults and Children. Hannover 1992 pp 26-32

25 Pinkerton CR, Williams D, Wooton C et al: 5HT3, antagonist ondansetron - an effective outpatient anti-emetic in cancer treatment. Arch Dis Child 1990 (65/8):822-825

26 Laupert A: The role of nurses in the nutrition and management of emesis in children with cancer. In: "Ondansetron" - Management of Emesis in Children with Cancer. Hannover 1992 pp 40-43

The Role of Nurses in the Prevention and Management of Emesis from Chemotherapy and Radiotherapy

Susie Wilkinson

Liverpool Marie Curie Cancer Centre, Speke Road, Woolton, Liverpool L25 8QA, United Kingdom

It has long since been established that cancer and its treatment can be a source of great distress for patients and their families. The time of diagnosis, as Greer remarked, is often viewed as a "catastrophic threat tantamount to a death sentence" [1]. Treatment is usually commenced soon after diagnosis and patients are then faced with the fear of death and the possible side-effects of treatment. While some patients are able to take the possibility of death stoically, many find the side-effects of treatment intolerable.

Chemotherapy is notorious for its side-effects. Several studies [2-4] have demonstrated that patients experience significant increases in anxiety and depression.

Emesis is perceived as the most distressing symptom associated with chemotherapy. It can even cause some patients to refuse, delay or discontinue treatment altogether [5,6]. Such decisions can create considerable stress to families and all those involved in patient care. Therefore, effective symptom management must be a priority for the health care team.

Nurses have most contact with patients and are the ones who best appreciate how much distress patients experience. In specialist units and in some general hospitals, nurses inform and prepare patients for the side-effects of chemotherapy and provide emotional support and encouragement to help them cope. They have perhaps been more aware than anyone else in the health care team of the significant problems emesis causes.

It is therefore not surprising that nursing patients with uncontrolled emesis has been identified as a major stressor for cancer nurses [7] and a survey of cancer nursing priorities [8] rated emesis as the area of nursing research that could have the greatest impact on nursing care. This chapter will focus on the care nurses can provide to help prevent and manage treatment-induced emesis.

The Nursing Management of Treatment-Induced Emesis

The impact of emesis can cause physical and psychological problems. Nausea and vomiting can range from a tolerable mild discomfort to serious complications such as nutritional deficits, dehydration, electrolyte imbalance, fatigue, weakness and gastrointestinal traumas [9]. These physical stresses are often compounded by psychological distress, such as anxiety and depression, which can lead to a severe disruption in life style.

The overall aim of nursing care should be directed towards enhancing a physiological/psychological well-being and preventing and minimising dehydration, weight loss and malnutrition. Nursing care needs to be based on detailed, individualised assessment.

Nursing Assessment

The nurse's role in assessment begins as soon as the patient is informed of the possibility of receiving treatment. Assessment can be divided into 3 areas:

a) general assessment;
b) treatment assessment;
c) emetic assessment.

General Assessment

This includes:

1. The history of present illness. How and when the patient first realised he had a problem, what he did about it and how he felt about it with precise details of any treatments to date.
2. The patient's awareness of diagnosis/prognosis. The patient's understanding of his diagnosis/prognosis and how he feels about it.
3. The history of previous illness. Brief details of previous illnesses and the physical and mental effects of them.
4. A physical assessment, including such areas as mobility, eliminations, respiration, skin, diet, allergies, medications and sleep, and the extent of the problems. Exactly how much or in what way has the problem affected the patient's normal, daily activities and how does the patient feel about this.
5. A social assessment, focussed on person(s) with whom the patient has a meaningful relationship, the extent of the support of and satisfaction with the relationship, patient's home conditions and ability to cope with household chores, patient's hobbies and leisure activities.
6. A psychological assessment of the patient's present mood state in terms of how the illness is affecting him. It is necessary to pick up on any cues of anxiety and depression and assess what impact the anxiety or depression has on the patient. In situations where the cancer is likely to disturb sexuality, e.g. cancer of the breast, colon, testes, sexual relationships need to be explored.

Treatment Assessment

Following the general assessment, a more detailed treatment assessment is valuable. This should focus on the patient's perception of the treatment and its side-effects. Exploration of what patients think may happen enables nurses to clarify any myths, false ideas or misconceptions.

Emetic Assessment

Taking into account the emetic potential of the prescribed treatment, the third part of the assessment needs to focus on the emetic susceptibility of the patient, including the predictors of anticipatory nausea and vomiting (ANV) [10] (Table 1) and factors which have been identified as affecting emesis [10] (Table 2).

It is also important to explore the patient's perception of nausea and vomiting as a problem. That is, what is an acceptable or unacceptable level of nausea and vomiting, prior experiences of nausea/vomiting and current or past coping strategies. The use of a formalised emesis assessment tool such as the form shown in Table 3 can be helpful [11]. Patient's interests in participating in alternative therapies known to help with emesis also need to be identified.

Time spent obtaining a detailed assessment is crucial as this serves as a basis for an accurate care plan. This time also enables nurses to form a relationship and partnership with patients. Nurses' assessment skills, however, remain very poor [12]. Most nurses' assessments have been shown to be very superficial

Table 1. Predictors of anticipated nausea and vomiting

* younger patients develop more ANV
* patients with a history of motion sickness develop more ANV
* unpleasant taste sensations during infusions increase ANV
* poorly controlled nausea and vomiting with prior chemotherapy increases ANV
* anxiety probably facilitates the development of ANV
* fear of venipuncture increases ANV

Table 2. Factors predisposing to increased emesis after chemotherapy

* women are more prone to vomiting than men
* younger patients vomit more
* a history of high alcohol intake reduces the emetic response
* susceptibility to motion sickness increases the emetic response
* emetic control is easier for the first treatment
* poor emetic control during previous treatment increases subsequent nausea and vomiting
* anxiety increases the emetic response
* antiemetic control is less efficient in outpatient settings

Table 3. A possible nausea and vomiting assessment tool

Patient ----------

Chemotherapy Regimen ----------

Antiemetic Regimen ----------

Have you experienced nausea/vomiting with illness, pregnancy, car sickness, etc? ----------

If so, was anything helpful to decrease this? ----------

Have you had nausea or vomiting with past chemotherapy? ----------

Was this tolerable or intolerable? ----------

What antinausea medicine did your doctor prescribe? ----------

Was it helpful? ----------

Did you take the medicine? ---------- How often? ----------

Did you have any side-effects with antinausea medicine? ----------

Do you think you will have vomiting from your chemotherapy? ----------

If the patient is receiving chemotherapy:

Are your experiencing nausea with your chemotherapy? ----------

When does it happen?(before,during,after) (onset) ----------

How long does it last? (duration) ----------

Rate your nausea in terms of intensity and interference with your life ---------- (use VAS scale)

Are you experiencing vomiting with your chemotherapy? ----------

When does it happen? (before,during,after) ----------

How long does it last? ----------

Rate your vomiting in terms of intensity and interference with your life ---------- (use VAS scale)

How satisfied are you with present control of nausea and/or vomiting? ----------

None at all VAS
Intolerable

0 ______________________________ 10

and few nurses appear to have the ability to evaluate accurately the physical problems patients experience and certainly not patients' mood states. Results of studies [12-14] indicate that in most areas and especially the areas of psychological care, nursing care often has been planned on assumption rather than data obtained from an assessment. Emesis related to chemo/radiotherapy will persist unnecessarily if nurses do not take the time and trouble to assess in depth the actual and potential problems patients may experience.

Education and Information

After assessment some patients require an explanation of the treatment and its possible side-effects. This is necessary as active seeking of information about cancer and its treatment has been identified as a coping mechanism to help patients gain control over their situation [15,16]. Recognising that information should be tailored to patients' needs, researchers have focussed on identifying the type of information cancer patients feel they need and when.

Derdiarian [17] conducted tape-recorded interviews with a convenience sample of 60 newly diagnosed cancer patients, using the Derdiarian Information Needs Assessment Schedule

(DINA). She found from an analysis of variance, that the following hierarchy of needs emerged in each of the 4 categories.

1. **Disease**	2. **Personal**
Treatment	Physical well-being
Prognosis	Psychological well-being
Diagnosis	Job/career
Tests	Plans/goals

3. **Family**	4. **Social relationships**
Spouse	Job
Children	Future
Parents	Leisure
Siblings	Special interests.

Significantly more people needed information about treatment (mean 46.0) than about any other category. More importance was given to treatment and prognosis (mean 44.0) than to diagnosis (mean 31.2) and tests (mean 26.1). The impact of cancer on physical and psychological well-being was more important than on jobs and plans. Women were more concerned about prognosis, psychological well-being and siblings. Those women with living parents also attached more importance to them and how to deal with their existing distress, compared with men who were more concerned about the diagnostic tests, their physical well-being and the effect on their spouse.

Younger adults (18-55) also needed more information on the possible effects their disease and treatment would have on their spouses, partners and careers. Patients with local disease needed more information than those with disseminated disease about the effects on their spouse.

Derdiarian concluded that although disease-related concerns are discussed more than personal, family or social concerns at the time of diagnosis, it is important for nurses to assess these other areas of concern on admission to hospital since they are frequently dismissed as not relevant. This highlights the fact that nurses should not assume what patients' needs are and should assess each patient's concerns individually.

Uncertainty about diagnosis and treatment appears to make patients more vulnerable to stress; this distress is often exacerbated by a failure to meet patients' informational needs. Doctors [18-20] and to some extent nurses [21] underestimate the amount and misperceive the type of information that is needed.

This misperception can result in patients seeking information through other channels, such as cues from the health carer's manner, examination, treatment and evasion when talking about the diagnosis [22]. Several studies [23,24] indicate that if patients are informed about their disease and treatment, this is beneficial in reducing anxiety and depression.

Nurses need to give a brief description of the actual treatment and a rough idea of how long it will take. They also need to indicate whether the chemotherapy will be given by infusions, injections or tablets, and whether the patient is likely to experience any physical symptoms. For example, if the treatment is given by infusion the patient may well feel a cold or warm sensation in the arm or some patients may experience a metallic taste in the mouth. If the chemotherapy regime is likely to produce delayed emesis, it is important to mention this as it could cause considerable distress to patients who were beginning to think they had survived chemotherapy without any vomiting. If patients are given a description of what they are likely to hear, feel, smell and taste, this enhances their ability to cope [25]. Radiotherapy patients can also experience nausea and vomiting due to high levels of anxiety or fear. A description of the radiotherapy machines with photographs or a visit to the unit with the assurance that although the patients may be left alone in the treatment room they will have contact with members of the staff, can do much to allay anxiety.

One study [26] evaluated a preparation package for patients receiving chemotherapy. The package consisted of a single 90-minute session held at the treatment centre before the first chemotherapy session. Family members were invited to join the patient during the session which consisted of 4 components:

1. the tour of the oncology unit and treatment area;
2. a video presentation of a chemotherapy treatment illustrating the procedure, providing information about a variety of common questions and showing a patient coping successfully with the treatment;
3. a question-and-answer period;
4. written material that summarised the information presented during the tour and videotape.

The results indicated that the preparation package increased patients' knowledge of the disease and its treatment, reduced nausea and vomiting, decreased negative effects and generally improved patients' coping ability.

While not all oncology units may be able to provide such in-depth preparation, any oral information given by nurses should be supplemented by written information so that patients and their carers can refer to it at a later stage. It is preferable that the written information is individualised to a particular hospital or unit. To help prepare information sheets or booklets it is perhaps worthwhile to obtain a published information booklet which is available in most countries from supporting organisations. In the UK such booklets can be obtained from Bacup*, Cancerlink** and The Royal Marsden***.

An alternative way of giving patients information which they can frequently refer to is by audiotape. As part of one of their annual awards The Royal College of Nursing, Cancer Nursing Society in England requested that nurses working in oncology units submit audiotapes that patients could receive prior to treatment, informing them about their treatment and its side-effects. Many tapes were submitted and are now in use in a large number of centres.

In summary, there are many ways of informing and educating patients about their disease, treatment and its side-effects. Whether it is by visits to the units, audiotapes, videotapes or written information, it now seems clear that as long as information is tailored to the patient's requirements, it has beneficial effects. One difficulty that nurses frequently experience in giving information to patients who request it, is the fear of getting into trouble with doctors. However, it has been shown that in oncology units where nurses have negotiated permission with doctors to inform patients about their disease or treatment if asked, communication between the nurses and patients is improved and a more relaxed ward environment is created [12]. The management of patient care is very much a team effort and it therefore is hoped that most nurses can obtain permission to give information to patients if they feel competent to do so. Whilst it is recognised that the amount of information patients receive regarding their diagnosis and treatment varies from country to country [27,28], it would appear from research undertaken in Western Europe and the United States that open communication has substantial benefits for patients.

Nursing Interventions

Physical Environment

For patients who are vomiting, a calm ward environment is important. The time of administering chemotherapy may influence patients' perception of emesis but not the actual occurrence [29]. Patients who receive chemotherapy during the evening reported less stress; this appeared to be related to the ability to relax in an environment that was less stimulating than that of patients being treated in the morning. Most importantly, patients treated at night estimated their nausea and vomiting to be less stressful than patients treated in the morning [29]. Privacy in a single room, or curtaining partitions for patients who want them, should always be available. In the outpatient setting, a patient satisfaction study [30] demonstrated that 80% of patients wanted privacy and they did not wish to have contact with other patients. It also concluded that comfortable armchairs rather that beds were preferable for receiving chemotherapy. Increased stress was experienced by patients if they had to wait for treatment and 71.4% of patients stated they would prefer their chemotherapy to be administered by the same nurse on each occasion, thus emphasising the importance of continuity of care.

Each patient needs access to a vomit bowl and tissues, mouth-care equipment, deodorisers, supplementary food and audiovisual equipment, if requested. Sights and smells often abound in hospital wards. Not only the sights and smells that are normally considered offensive matter: what to one person is a delicious aroma may be extremely nauseating to another. Patients who feel nauseous or inclined to vomiting need to be kept away from areas

---

* BACUP (British Association of Cancer United Patients), 3 Bath Place, Rivington Street, London EC2A 3JR, Tel. 0800 181199

** Cancerlink, 17 Britannia Street, London WCX 9JN, Tel. +44 171 8332451

*** The Royal Marsden Hospital, Downs Road, Sutton, Surrey SM2 5PT, Tel. +44 181 6426011

where food is prepared or eaten. Not only the sights and smells associated with food may cause emesis; in an oncology ward malodorous wounds can act as a vomiting stimulus. Odorous fungating tumours, for example, are very difficult to control. Preparations such as metronidazole gel and activated charcoal dressings can be applied to reduce odour. Other preparations which disguise or neutralise the smell are available but a major problem with some of these preparations and many other hospital disinfectants is that they have a very distinctive smell which may also become a vomiting stimulus.

Monitoring Emesis

If nausea and vomiting are to be successfully controlled, a team approach is important. Due to their frequent contact with patients, nurses have a specific role in monitoring the response to treatment. Fitch [31] recommends that nurses monitor patients to ensure that:

a) sufficient antiemetic is administered at the onset of treatment to prevent the experience of nausea and vomiting;
b) antiemetics are administered regularly rather than on an "as needed" basis;
c) where antiemetics are not effective, doctors are informed to enable the implementation of alternative treatments;
d) adequate antiemetic coverage is in place for delayed emesis.

Whether emesis is monitored by observation or diaries, nurses have a responsibility to inform doctors of their findings. Patients, whether in hospital or in the community, can be taught to keep a diary to record information about their vomiting and its impact on their daily living and physical condition. An example of a tool that can be used to monitor the effectiveness of antiemetic therapy is the INV/2 questionnaire [32]. This is an 8-item, 5-point Likert-type self-report tool that was developed to measure how patients perceive the duration, frequency and distress of nausea, the frequency and distress of vomiting and of dry heaves. A total score on the INV/2 provides the patient's total experience score. The questionnaire also captures the differences between the actual occurrences of vomiting and the emotional response that the patient associates with his symptoms; it has been used in several nursing studies [33-35].

Non-Pharmacological Management of Emesis

Mouth Care

The nurse's role also involves providing several practical non-pharmacological supportive measures which include mouth care. Oral hygiene is important for patient comfort and prevention of infection which, in immunosuppressed patients, can have severe complications. Regular mouth care, especially after patients have vomited, is vital as it removes debris from the mouth, thus reducing the chance of infection. The choice of mouthwash necessitates careful consideration as some patients find the taste of preparatory mouthwashes nauseating. Some patients may only be able to tolerate rinsing their mouth with ice-cold water or with water and sodium bicarbonate, which may not be as effective as a preparatory mouthwash; however, if this does not induce vomiting, it is better than nothing. In patients who have lost weight it is not unusual to encounter ill-fitting dentures which can lead to sore mouths, difficulty with eating, retching and vomiting. The help of a dentist should be enlisted as simply re-lining the dentures may solve the problem.

Dietary Factors

Flexibility has to be an integral part of any care plan for patients who experience emesis. This can prove to be difficult in busy wards. The provision of small, attractively served meals when the patient wants to eat is important. A free choice of diet, enabling patients to avoid foods which they feel could induce further nausea and vomiting, is necessary. Patients are often asked to choose meals the day before they eat them and when they arrive it is usually at a set time. In general the meals have been already plated, with all 3 courses served on the same tray; this can be very off-putting. Very little time and effort is necessary to offer courses separately, but these difficulties often arise because meals are served by catering staff who cannot or are not expected to know how much patients would like to eat. Because of these problems it is preferable that dieticians and the catering staff are involved when care is being planned for patients who are likely to experience emesis. If patients do not want their meal at the time it arrives on the ward, provision to store meals until a more suitable time is necessary. Dietary advice to patients with taste aberrations can often make food more acceptable and less nauseating; for example, patients who have a distaste for sweetness can benefit from increased seasoning or flavouring in their food, for some patients drinking cold fizzy drinks and sucking ice can reduce nausea.

Dehydration

If patients are unable to eat, small frequent drinks, even if it is only water, are necessary to avoid dehydration. Monitoring for early signs and symptoms of dehydration (Table 4) is essential [36]. If dehydration is suspected, the doctor needs to be informed immediately.

Psychological Support

As well as monitoring and providing interventions for physical symptoms associated with emesis, the nurse also has a role in monitoring psychological distress and providing psychological support.

Patients may experience several fears when faced with a course of chemotherapy or radiotherapy including:

1) fear of the disease;
2) fear of the unknown;
3) fear of not coping with the treatment;
4) fear of losing control;
5) fear of being abandoned.

In order to alleviate such fears nurses need to facilitate discussion of them; however, research indicates that many nurses find this very difficult [12-14]. In order to help patients, nurses

Table 4. Symptoms relating to the loss of body fluid

Loss of total body fluid (%)	Symptom or clinical manifestation
2%-4%	Thirst
Mild-moderate dehydration	
2.5%-5%	Dryness of tongue Scanty or decreased urine output High urine specific gravity Furrowed tongue Decreased turgidity of skin Elevated BUN
5%-8%	Fatique Increased pulse Elevated temperature Deterioration of mental processes
Serious dehydration	
6%-10%	Protein, casts and erythrocytes excreted in urine Loss of skin turgor
Severe dehydration	
10%	Sunken eyeballs Profound depression Anuria 10% increase in haematocrit
11%-15%	Delirium Deafness Kidney failure
10%-20%	Death

Table 5. Required communication skills

Listening
Acknowledging
Open questions
Picking up of cues
Reflection
Clarification
Encouragement
Empathy

need to master several communication skills as shown in Table 5.

If patients are distressed it is important to allow them to describe how they are feeling. Listening is not easy, it takes great concentration and it is not a skill most doctors and nurses are good at [36]. One reason for poor listening is that while patients talk, most doctors and nurses start to think about how they are going to respond. This results in the last part of what patients say (which may include vital cues) being missed. To demonstrate listening is taking place, acknowledgement is necessary, for example, nodding or saying "yes" or "right". To encourage patients to talk about how they are feeling, reflection is an effective technique, for example, patient: "I am really worried about this"; response: "You're really worried". Patients often then continue to discuss how they are feeling. It is not enough to know patients are worried, it is necessary to explore exactly what patients are worrying about. For this, open questions allowing open responses from patients are necessary. For example, "What exactly is worrying you at the present moment?" Sometimes it is necessary to find out more details about patients' worries and the skill to use is clarification. For example, patient: "I'm very worried about receiving chemotherapy." Response: "Could you possibly tell me exactly what part of the chemotherapy you are worried about?" Occasionally when patients talk about worries or concerns it becomes obvious they need encouragement and help to continue, for example, "That's very interesting, could you possibly bear to tell me just a little bit more about that?" Empathy is a skill which is rarely used by nurses [12]; it is, however, one of the most unobtrusive and effective skills for facilitating exploration of feelings. Empathy demonstrates recognition that what patients are experiencing or are feeling is very difficult. For example, "From what you've just told me it really sounds as if what you are going through is awful." Empathy in no way minimises the situation or the extent of the patient's feelings.

There are, however, several verbal behaviours which block patients from talking about how they feel. These behaviours are rarely helpful to patients [12-14,37]. Patients are often reluctant to disclose exactly how they feel for fear of being considered stupid, and if their feelings are greeted with responses as shown in Table 6, they will on future occasions be even more reluctant.

Table 6. Blocking verbal behaviours

Patient: "I'm so anxious I am really finding this vomiting so difficult to cope with"	
Changing topic	"Are you having any visitors today?"
Normalising stereotyped	"I know it's very difficult we see a lot of this the whole time"
False premature reassurance	"Oh, don't worry about it you'll be through it soon, it will all be alright in the end"
Passing the buck	"Have you told the doctor how awful you feel?"
Jollying along	"Don't look so glum about it, it'll all be alright, please give me a smile"
Inappropriate advising	"You'll continue to feel like this I am afraid for this course of chemotherapy and of course in the next one you will probably also feel like this again, but we will try somehow to make you feel a little bit better"
Change of focus to relative	"Have you told your wife how awful you are feeling"

The kind of responses patients require at times of distress are empathic responses. Whatever feeling is experienced - it may be fear, worry, anxiety - it can be responded to by using the following guidelines:

- recognition of non-verbal or verbal anxiety;
- acknowledgement - "I can see you are anxious";
- permission - "It's OK for you to be anxious";
- understanding - "I want to find out what is making you anxious";
- empathic acceptance - "You are anxious because... ";
- assessment - severity and effects of anxiety;
- alteration (if appropriate);
- removal of stress;
- cognitive challenge;
- boosting coping strategies;
- medication.

Such techniques give patients permission to express how they are feeling and hope that their difficulties will be taken seriously and that attempts will be made to improve the situation. This may not always be possible. One study, however, has demonstrated that when patients were facilitated to tell the doctor how they were feeling even though there was not a solution to their problems, their levels of anxiety were significantly reduced [38]. This emphasises that one of the most important roles nurses have is to allow patients to talk about how they feel as this may help them cope better with the nausea and vomiting they may experience.

Other methods of monitoring how patients are coping with treatment are quality-of-life tools. Before using a quality-of-life assessment tool it is important to liaise with the entire health care team, and especially the doctors, to see that this form of monitoring is acceptable. There are many available which have been reviewed by Fallowfield [39]. One of the tools that are easy for nurses to administer is the Hospital Anxiety and Depression scale (HADS) [40]. The HADS scale consists of 14 items, 7 for each subscale, and patients rate items on a 4-point scale. The scale was developed to measure the levels of anxiety and depression in hospital patients. It is very quick to administer, complete and score, and therefore acceptable to patients. Two other instruments which focus not just on psychological aspects but also on physical symptoms, functional and quality-of-life status are the Rotterdam Symptom Checklist (RSCL) [41] and the EORTC Quality of Life Questionnaire 30, version 2.0 [42]. Patients can complete these before and after chemotherapy, thus assessing how they are coping from their own perspective. A quality-of-life assessment tool can also be used to identify patients who might benefit from alternative therapies.

Alternative Therapies

Alternative therapies which nurses can apply and which have been shown to be beneficial to patients include distraction, relaxation and guided imagery, massage/aromatherapy, aerobics and acupressure. The choice of therapies is best discussed with patients and initiated before treatment begins, as interventions appear to have the most effect when introduced early in the treatment process; however, if they are introduced after treatment is commenced, they can still have some effect [26].

Distraction

With guidance, patients can learn to use distraction techniques such as computer games, watching television or listening to music. In a comprehensive study [26] simple distraction techniques, when compared with other alternative therapies, proved to be very cost-effective and a successful way of preventing and controlling emesis.

Relaxation

More than any other technique, behavioural relaxation procedures, especially progressive muscle relaxation training followed by guided imagery, have been shown to reduce the distress of chemotherapy [26]. Nurses are in a good position to undertake progressive muscle relaxation training with patients. It is important that the first session is audiotaped so that patients can keep the tape and use it on other occasions. This also has the benefit for patients of hearing a voice they know and are familiar with. Once patients have completed the muscle tensing and relaxing procedures, they can be provided with several minutes of a relaxing imagery consisting of a sequence of thoughts or mental pictures that facilitate deeper relaxation. The kind of image that patients find relaxing will differ individually and this can be determined by the pre-treatment discussion. Patients can then be encouraged to practise the relaxation frequently, especially during the days immediately following chemotherapy when the side-effects tend to be most severe. This form of alternative therapy has proved to be successful in several studies [43-46].

Massage/Aromatherapy

If nurses are in possession of a recognised training in massage techniques, gentle body massage has also proved to be very successful in relaxing patients [47,48]. The massage can be performed either with or without an essential oil. If aromatherapy oils are used, the smell of the oil must be acceptable to the patient. Gentle massage in a darkened room with soft music can greatly enhance the patient's feeling of well-being.

Aerobics

There is some initial evidence [49] suggesting that regular individualised aerobic exercise routines reduce nausea for some patients undergoing chemotherapy if the aerobic exercise is carried out 3 times a week, over a period of weeks; however, further research is needed to substantiate these findings.

Acupressure

Acupressure bands, or seabands as they are sometimes called, can be helpful for some patients. These are elasticated wrist bands with a button that presses on the P6 Neiguan pressure point, believed to affect the vomiting centre. Two small studies [50,51] have demonstrated that with the use of these bands some nausea remained but it was greatly reduced, fluids and diet were better tolerated, and patients felt that they were more in control of their care and consequently experienced less anxiety and depression.

Nurse Education

To enable nurses to provide optimum care for patients experiencing emesis, they need education in cancer care. There is evidence suggesting that few nurses in their general training receive adequate education in caring for cancer patients [52,53]. Furthermore, results of an international study indicate [54] that nurses in most countries have not received sufficient education and training in the management of emesis, causing them to feel stressed [7]. Conversely, nurses who have completed post-basic education in cancer nursing, which includes the management of emesis, feel more competent and able to help patients in discussing their worries and concerns [12]. Whilst post-basic courses are not available in many countries, three recent initiatives may prove helpful for improving the education of nurses in this area. The first is an educational package designed jointly by the International Society of Nurses in Cancer Care and Glaxo Laboratories. This package focusses specifically on the nursing care of patients who experience vomiting induced by chemotherapy and radiotherapy [55]. The second initiative is the Diploma in Cancer Care, a Distance Learning Programme produced by the Marie Curie Cancer Care Foundation* and accredited by the Humberside College of Nursing.

This distance learning programme enables nurses to learn about cancer and its treatments. On receiving the learning materials, nurses are able to work through the programme at their own pace. Assessment of learning incorporates assignments and a final examination.

The third initiative, Cancer Care Priorities for Nurses, is a European Oncology Nursing Society educational programme sponsored by a grant from SmithKline Beecham and coordinated by Cooney Waters Interscience**. Nurses from European countries met to draw up educational booklets containing guidelines and model curricula for teaching 5 areas of cancer care: Altered Body Image, Emesis, Psychological Disorders, Pain and Infections. Nurses throughout

* Cancer Care Nursing Diploma, Marie Curie Cancer Care, Education Department, 11 Lyndhurst Gardens, Hampstead, London NW3 5NS, U.K.

** Cooney Waters Interscience, Aldwych House, 81 Aldwych, London WC2B 4DB, U.K. Tel. +44 171 404 2074, Fax +44 171 331 0333

Europe interested in this programme should contact Cooney Waters Interscience.

Conclusion

Nurses, who provide 24-hour care to patients, have a unique role to play in the prevention and management of emesis from chemo/radiotherapy. Assessment data of a patient's physical and psychological needs and susceptibility to vomiting must be routinely shared with doctors to ensure patients receive the most effective antiemetic therapy before treatment commences, also to avoid anticipatory emesis. Nurses have an important role in making sure that prescribed antiemetics are given at the correct time and patients do not have to wait or ask for their antiemetic drugs. Patients who are informed about their treatment and disease appear to cope better with emesis than patients who have not been fully informed. Therefore nurses, who have most contact with patients, have a duty to keep patients up-to-date with all the information they require. For patients who do experience emesis, nurses have the responsibility to ensure the physical environment minimises the risk of further nausea and vomiting. Nurses also have an important task in providing psychological support to patients. This requires good communication skills which include being able to respond to patients empathically. Finally, nurses are in a good position to give alternative therapies. As with antiemetic drugs these therapies seem to be most effective if they are commenced before the start of treatment. Knowledgeable nurses are able to give better care and there is evidence suggesting that nurses in the 1990s do not find patients undergoing chemotherapy as stressful as previous research reported [56]. This is thought to be due to new antiemetic drugs and improved antiemetic regimes.

It would appear that in the opinion of nurses [56], emesis associated with radio/chemotherapy is improving for patients in oncology units but for patients treated in general hospitals improvements will only become apparent if both doctors and nurses receive comprehensive education in the prevention and management of chemo/radiotherapy-induced emesis.

REFERENCES

1 Greer S: Cancer; psychiatric aspects. In: Granville-Grossman K (ed) Recent Advances in Clinical Psychiatry. Churchill Livingstone, London 1985

2 Maguire P, Tait A, Brooke M, Sellwood R: Emotional aspects of mastectomy. Planning a caring programme. Nursing Mirror 1980 (150/17):35-37

3 Hughes JE: Psychological and social consequences of cancer. Cancer Surv 1987 (6):455-475

4 Hughson AVM, Cooper AF: The Psychological impact of adjuvant chemotherapy following mastectomy. In: Watson M, Greer S, Thomas C (eds) Psychosocial Oncology. Pergamon Press, Oxford 1988 pp 101-110

5 Love RR, Leventhal H, Easterling DV: Side effects and emotional distress during cancer chemotherapy. Cancer 1989 (63):604-612

6 Laszlo J: Nausea and vomiting as major complications of cancer chemotherapy. Drugs 1983 (25 Suppl 1):1-7

7 Wilkinson SM: The satisfaction and stresses of nursing cancer patients. Unpublished M.Sc. Thesis, University of Manchester 1986

8 Oberst MT: Priorities in cancer nursing research. Cancer Nursing 1978 (1):281-290

9 Enck RE: Mallory-Weiss lesion following cancer chemotherapy. Lancet 1979 (Oct 29):927-928

10 Hawthorn J: Can we predict post-chemotherapy nausea and vomiting? Int Cancer Nursing News 1993 (5):9

11 Wickham R: Managing chemotherapy-related nausea and vomiting: The state of the art. Oncology Nursing Forum 1989 (16):563-574

12 Wilkinson SM: Factors which influence how nurses communicate with cancer patients. J Adv Nursing 1991 (16):677-688

13 Bond S: Processes of communication about cancer in a radiotherapy department. Unpublished Ph D Thesis, University of Edinburgh 1978

14 Faulkner A: Communication of information to patients. In: Faulkner A (ed) Recent Advances in Nursing Communication, Vol 7. Churchill Livingstone, Edinburgh 1984

15 Weisman AD: Coping with Cancer. McGraw Hill, New York 1979

16 Friedman BD: Coping with cancer: a guide for health care professionals. Cancer Nursing 1980 (2):105-110

17 Derdiarian A: Informational needs of recently diagnosed cancer patients. Nursing Res 1986 (36):276-281

18 Faden RR, Becker C, Lewis C, Freeman J, Faden AI: Disclosure of information to patients. Med Care 1981 (7):718-733

19 Laver P, Murphy SP, Powers MJ: Learning needs of cancer patients; a comparison of nurse and patient perception. Nursing Res 1982 (5):11-16

20 Messerli ML, Garamendi C, Romano J: Breast cancer; information as a technique crisis intervention. Am J Ortho-Psychiatry 1980 (50):728-731

21 Frank-Stromborg M, Wright P: Ambulatory cancer patients' perception of physical and psychosocial changes in their lives since a diagnosis of cancer. Cancer Nursing 1984 (7):117-130

22 Slevin M: Talking about cancer; how much is too much? Br J Hosp Med 1987 (38):56-59

23 Hames A, Stirling E: Choice aids recovery. Nursing Times 1987 (83):49-51

24 Morris J, Royle GT: Choice of surgery for early breast cancer: pre and postoperative levels of clinical anxiety and depression in patients and their husbands. Br J Surgery 1987 (15):429-434

25 Strohl RA: The nursing role in radiation oncology: symptom management of acute and chronic reactions. Oncol Nursing Forum 1988 (15):429-434

26 Burish TG, Tope DM: Psychological techniques for controlling the adverse side effects of cancer chemotherapy: findings from a decade of research. J Pain & Symptom Management 1992 (7):287-301

27 Zwitter M, Williams CJ: Informed consent in European multicentric randomised clinical trials. Eur J Cancer 1993 (29A Suppl 6):S212

28 Pronzato P, Losardo PL, Cantinotti E, Colombo F, Dal Mut D, Pacolini L, Scopsi G, Bertelli G, Ospedale S Andrea, La Spezia and National Institute for Cancer Research, Genova, Italy: Knowledge of diagnosis in Italian patients with advanced cancer. Eur J Cancer 1993 (29A Suppl 6):S212

29 Headley JA: The influence of administration time on chemotherapy-induced nausea and vomiting. Oncol Nursing Forum 1987 (14):43-47

30 Rudbaek H, Thy U, Sand D: The influence of the hospital environment for the outpatient receiving chemotherapy. Eur J Cancer 1993 (29A Suppl 6):S256

31 Fitch MJ: Managing treatment-induced emesis: A nursing perspective. Oncology 1992 (49):312-316

32 Rhodes VA, Watson PM, Johnson MH: Development of reliable and valid measures of nausea and vomiting. Cancer Nursing 1984 (7):33-41

33 Troesch LM, Blust Rodehaver C, Delaney EA, Yanes B: The influence of guided imagery on chemotherapy-related nausea and vomiting. Oncol Nursing Forum 1993 (20):1179-1185

34 Rhodes VA, Watson PM, Johnson MH, Madsen RW, Beck NC: Patterns of nausea, vomiting and distress in patients receiving antineoplastic drug protocols. Oncol Nursing Forum 1987 (14):35-44

35 Nolan EM: Nausea, vomiting and dehydration. In: Jacobs M and Geels W (eds) Signs and Symptoms in Nursing: Interpretation and Management. Lippincott & Co, Philadelphia 1985

36 Maguire P, Rutter DR: History taking for medical students. Deficiencies in performance. Lancet 1976 (2):556-558

37 Quint JC: The Nurse and the Dying Patient. Macmillan, New York 1967

38 Macleod R: Patients with advanced breast cancer: The nature and disclosure of their concerns. Unpublished M.Sc. Thesis, University of Manchester 1992

39 Fallowfield L: The Quality of Life, The Missing Measurement In Health Care. Souvenir Press, London 1990

40 Zigmond A, Snaith R: The hospital anxiety and depression scale. Acta Psychiatr Scand 1983 (67): 361-370

41 De Haes JCJM, Knippenberg FCE, Neijt JP: Measuring psychological and physical distress in can-

cer patients: Structure and application of the Rotterdam Symptom checklist. Br J Cancer 1990 (62): 1034-1038
42 Aaronson NK et al: The European Organization for Research and Treatment of Cancer QLQ-30: A quality-of-life instrument for use in international clinical trials in oncology. JNCI 1993 (85):5
43 Warren K: Will I be sick, nurse? Nursing Times 1988 (12):30-32
44 Troesch LM, Blust Rodehaver C, Delaney E, Yanes B: The influence of guided therapy on chemotherapy related nausea and vomiting. Oncol Nursing Forum 1993 (20):1179-1185
45 Redd W, Andrykowski M: Behavioural interventions in cancer treatment controlling aversion reactions to chemotherapy. J Consult Clin Psycholgy 1982 (50): 1018-1029
46 Pervan V: Practical aspects of dealing with cancer therapy induced nausea and vomiting. Sem Oncol Nursing 1990 (6):3-5
47 Corner J, Cawley N, Hilderbrand S: An evaluation of the use of massage and essential oils on the wellbeing of cancer patients. Int J Palliat Nurs 1995 (1):2
48 Wilkinson S: Aromatherapy and massage in palliative care. Int J Palliat Nurs 1995 (1):1
49 Winningham ML, MacVicar MG: The effect of aerobic exercise on patient reports of nausea. Oncol Nursing Forum 1988 (15):447-450
50 Stannard D: Pressure prevents nausea. Nursing Times 1989 (85):33-34
51 Price H, Lewithg Williams C: Accupressure as an anti-emetic in chemotherapy. Compl Med Res 1991 (5):93-94
52 Corner J, Wilson-Barnett J: The newly-registered nurse and the cancer patient: an educational evaluation. Int J Nursing Studies 1992 (29):177-180
53 Copp K: Education and training in cancer - a European perspective. Cancer Nursing 1986 (11):255-258
54 Pritchard AP, Speechley V: What do nurses know about emesis? Int Cancer News 1984 (1):1
55 Hawthorn J: The management of nausea and vomiting induced by chemotherapy and radiotherapy. International Training Package for Nurses, Glaxo Holdings PLC 1991
56 Wilkinson S: The changing pressures of cancer nurses 1986-1993. Eur J Cancer 1995 (4):69-74

Evaluating the Cost-Effectiveness of New Drugs: the "Setrons" as an Example

Volker Kirchner [1] and Matti S. Aapro [2]

1 Division of Cell Biology, Harvard Medical School, and Division of Signal Transduction, Beth Israel Hospital, Alpert Building, 1st Floor, 200 Longwood Avenue, Boston, MA 02115, U.S.A.

2 Divisione di Oncologia Medica, Istituto Europeo di Oncologia, via Ripamonti 435, 20141 Milano, Italy, and Division d'Onco-Hématologie, Hôpital Cantonal Universitaire, 1211 Genève, Switzerland

Therapeutic innovations inevitably have an impact on treatment budgets. Since the introduction of 5-HT_3 receptor antagonists ("setrons"), the antiemetic budget has increased eight-fold from 1990 to 1992, which corresponds to an increase of 8% to 30% in the drug costs of hospital pharmacies [1]. This suggests the need for economic analyses especially as health-care resources are limited and hospital policy makers have to make difficult choices in a climate of cost containment. Cost is not merely a currency transaction but reflects the consumption of a resource that could otherwise be used for another purpose.

Why is this debate particularly relevant in the area of setrons? This family of antiemetic drugs seems ideal. They are safe through a very large dosing range, are not schedule-dependent and are effective in most patients over a wide dose range [2]. Indeed, the pharmacopoeia improved considerably with the introduction of the setrons.

But this advance is perceived as debatable since emesis is usually not considered as a life-threatening symptom and supportive care therapy still has to struggle to get quality of life studies considered as hard data. The question becomes: Is the treatment worth the money? In addition, other factors are responsible for inappropriate medication usage and unnecessary costs. First, there remains confusion about cancer-related emesis and the associated syndromes, such as acute nausea or vomiting or anticipatory nausea and vomiting or delayed nausea and vomiting. The implications of the defined syndromes are not understood, at least not in the general medical community, and this leads to an abuse of the setrons. Secondly, even if chemotherapy schedules have been classified according to their emetogenic potential, they convey confounding factors not only for the assessment of antiemetic studies, but especially in clinical practice. The same cytotoxic drug can be administered in various ways: single-day treatment versus fractionated chemotherapy over up to 5 days; oral or intravenous; direct intravenous injection or continuous intravenous infusion. All these modalities change the emetogenicity of the chemotherapy. Thirdly, regulatory agencies have approved the indications of setrons in anticancer cytotoxic treatment, but the registered doses and treatment schedules may vary between countries, as has been shown with ondansetron and granisetron. Once a higher dosage has been recommended it becomes hard to switch to lower doses, as we have seen with ondansetron [3]. Finally, the label of some commercially available oral setrons suggests continuous prescription up to 5 days after administration of chemotherapy, despite the disputed role of the setrons in late emesis.

Before any economic evaluation can be conducted 3 questions need to be addressed: 1) What kind of study should be chosen to conduct a clinical economic evaluation?; 2) At what point should an economic analysis be done?; and 3) Do the costs have a wider implication for medical research?

* This paper is based on a presentation given at the European Winter Oncology Conference (EWOC), Meribel, France, 1993

Clinical Economic Evaluation

The undertaking of economic analyses alongside clinical trials has never been a clear-cut matter [4-8]. Clinical trials are recognised as the best source of data for efficacy, but the care given during the trial may be so atypical that it is perhaps unwise to extrapolate these data to evaluate the economic impact of a new drug in normal practice [9]. Thus, a standard clinical trial design results in substantial interference with the normal pattern of patient management. This is essential if clinical trials are to answer therapeutic questions in a scientific manner but limits their usefulness in assessing the costs and benefits of therapy under conditions of normal usage. However, an assessment of the price and recommended usage of an innovation can give an indication of the potential cost of a compound. In practice, if there is a wide range of recommended usage or if an innovation is used indiscriminately, the costs can be substantially greater than estimates based upon recommended usage. Pragmatic clinical studies that assess the impact of therapy in a cohort of patients while keeping protocol driven interference to a minimum could provide an alternative to measuring the cost-effectiveness of new therapies.

Pragmatic Clinical Studies Versus Standard Clinical Trials

Two broad questions are useful in interpreting the results of a trial: Can the treatment work under ideal circumstances and does it work in ordinary settings? In this context, the distinction between efficacy and effectiveness needs to be outlined.

Efficacy is established by restricting patients in a study to those who will cooperate fully with medical advice. It is an evaluation of a treatment under ideal conditions. These are "equalised", "optimal" or "laboratory" conditions for a standard clinical trial, an explanatory or an intention-to-treat trial. It could be a randomised study or a cohort study. The aim here is to acquire information.

Effectiveness is established by offering a treatment or programme to patients under "ordinary" or "normal" conditions in what is called a pragmatic trial. It is a management trial and could be used to study cost-effectiveness. The aim here is to make a decision [10-14].

It is interesting to examine some differences between common practice and clinical trials. A major aim of common practice trials is external validity or generalisability and the relief of symptoms, whereas a clinical efficacy study is concerned with the internal validity of the clinical endpoint. The objectives of the two kinds of trials are quite different. Common practice requires a realistic estimate of drug impact, whereas clinical trials require control of the confounding variable or the "drug effect". The study design for these two situations is quite different, as discussed above. The comparisons made will also be quite different. In trials of common practice, a comparison is inevitably made with current practice, whereas in clinical trials the comparison is usually with placebo or therapeutic gold standards. The kinds of patients entered in these trials are also quite different. In common practice, comparisons are made with "everyday patients", whereas in clinical trials they are made with a highly selected group. In terms of evaluation, data are thought to be "soft" in common practice trials because symptom relief and quality of life are being evaluated and "hard" in clinical trials because a well defined endpoint like survival is the key goal.

The various theoretical requirements explain some biases of standard clinical trials and may contribute to some differences with pragmatic trials [15-19]. In any clinical trial, a clinician first selects a sample of people at risk, which is then randomised. The sample is then exposed (or not) to a drug and the outcome measured. In this process it is possible to introduce bias in sampling, selection and measurement.

Data from the Coronary Artery Surgery Study (CASS) exemplify the problem clearly [17]. This study was a randomised trial comparing clinical versus medical treatment in patients with stable coronary artery disease. Initially 16,626 patients were potentially eligible for the study. After all the normal exclusion criteria had been applied, only 12.7% of patients were suitable for entry into the study. When the inclusion/exclusion criteria as specified in the study protocol were applied, only 4.7% of patients were eligible for randomisation [20,21].

A clinician usually makes a diagnosis at the appearance of the first significant symptom for the patient. When conducting a trial, the clinician makes regular evaluations which will allow the detection of symptoms to be made early on and to be treated quite differently, especially when the clinical outcome would have been spontaneously favourable, which is in marked contrast to common practice [22].

In the case of adverse-event analysis, it is known that liver enzyme abnormalities, for example, are an adverse event which has been associated with 5-HT_3 receptor antagonists and chemotherapy [23-25]. This is only detected through blood sampling and has no clinical relevance, its detection serves merely to increase the indirect costs of the treatment [26, 27].

To summarise, clinical trials are not the best way to conduct a clinical economic evaluation. However, they are all that is available at present. Clinical trials do not necessarily address the problem of cost evaluation but when cost considerations are essential, it becomes crucial to determine the implications of cost evaluation in a clinical trial at an early stage.

Cost Studies

In order to assess the economic efficiency of a particular new treatment, it is necessary to examine its effect in three areas. Firstly, the impact on health service resources (hospital and ambulatory cost, pharmacist, medical and nursing time, equipment, drugs, etc.). Secondly, one should examine the impact on other community resources (input from patients and families, patient's ability to work). Finally, one needs to examine the impact of the new therapy on health status by evaluating improvements in health *per se* and in terms of other effects including money, health effects such as lives saved, or health "utilities" such as quality-adjusted life years [19].

An economic analysis can be represented in three dimensions [19,28-34]. Firstly, it is necessary to consider the types of analysis: cost identification (enumeration of costs involved in medical care ignoring the outcome of treatment), cost benefit (comparison of the management strategies in which the costs and benefits are both expressed in the same terms) or cost effectiveness (comparison of management strategies in terms of their cost per unit of output, where output is an outcome such as additional years of life, utilities, or additional cases of newly detected disease). Secondly, it is important to consider from which point of view the conclusions will be drawn, i.e., the patient, the payer, the provider or society. Thirdly, the type of costs must be considered and it is important to ensure that all have been taken into account:

- Direct costs: resources required to produce a service. These stem from transactions for goods or services, and include physician, drug, and direct non-medical costs such as those paid for by patients and their families. These costs can be variable, increasing with increasing volume of activity, or be fixed.
- Indirect costs: those which do not stem from transactions for goods or services. Costs of mortality and morbidity.
- Intangible costs: those of pain, suffering, and grief. These are usually extremely difficult to measure and often omitted in clinical economic research.

Antiemetic Cost Studies

Antiemetic cost studies have been carried out looking mainly at highly emetogenic chemotherapy regimens in an inpatient setting. An exception is the study by Cox [35], which is a retrospective analysis in an outpatient setting using cyclophosphamide-based chemotherapy. The majority of trials conducted so far are retrospective cost analyses, involving small numbers of patients. All ondansetron trials except for the Sands study used high-dose ondansetron (24-32 mg given as 3 or 4 divided doses i.v.) [11,12,36]. In comparative studies with granisetron, however, up to 80% of patients were treated with a single daily dose of 3 mg [36,37]. This simplified treatment regimen with granisetron is supposed to reduce direct costs of antiemetic therapy associated with drug acquisition, nursing time and materials necessary for the drug's administration. These elements have been discussed as relevant in drug cost-effectiveness analyses [38,39]. A sensitivity analysis has been carried out for two studies [11,38] with an analysis based on a decision analytic framework. The type of costs considered and the perspectives taken are not the same in these studies. Costs presented are based on the UK health-care system (ondansetron-based studies) or the Swiss health-care system (granisetron-based studies) and may vary between countries. The costs of non-proprietary brands of standard drugs may affect their acquisition cost, although in the UK the costs of intravenous generic brands are the same as those of the proprietary brands. Some of the non-drug costs associated with the two antiemetics (such as inpatient stays, cost of staff time for administering the drugs and the numerous tests associated with cytotoxic treatment) will fall under other budgets. The time spent by a nurse or a physician may diminish with the use of more efficient antiemetic drugs, but the staff costs will remain the same, as they are fixed [8,32,40-44]. Labour, materials and hospital stay can vary between institutions. In addition, since these data were published the costs of 5-HT_3 receptor antagonist drugs have been significantly reduced. All these changes can affect an economic evaluation and should be kept in mind [45]. In general these studies highlight the fact that decisions made purely on the narrow basis of drug costs may mislead decision makers and promote inefficient use of health resources [28].

Cost of Ondansetron Versus Metoclopramide in Acute Emesis

The impact of chemotherapy-associated nausea and vomiting on patients' functional status and cost has been prospectively evaluated before the commercial introduction of this particular 5-HT_3 serotonin-receptor antagonist. This impact has been a significant worsening of the functional status, a total cost of 184 Canadian dollars and disruption of the patients' close environment [46]. The study by Cunningham et al. [12] was an open, multicentre, randomised, parallel-group, unblinded study involving 2 centres. Thirty-two patients were randomised to receive either ondansetron (8 mg intravenously 4 hours for 3 doses) or metoclopramide (3 mg/kg i.v. loading dose, followed by 0.5 mg/kg/h i.v. for 8 hours). Nursing staff recorded the number of emetic episodes, details of adverse events, and specific data related to direct costs of antiemetic treatment such as all materials used in the administration of the antiemetic and time spent caring for the patient. No significant emesis was defined as one or less emetic episode during the 24-hour period following chemotherapy with no adverse events. Drug costs were derived from the Monthly Index of Medical Specialties (February 1991) and the British National Formulary No 19 (April 1990). Average staff wages were determined using data from the Department of Health, and material costs were based on Health Service Costing Returns 1986/89. Successful treatment was achieved in 50% of ondansetron-treated patients (7/14) and in 22% of metoclopramide-treated patients (4/18). The drug cost of ondansetron in the first 24 hours following chemotherapy was approximately 4 times greater than that of metoclopramide (£44.57 versus £11.91 per patient). The mean utilisation cost (considering the direct cost) was 2.5-fold higher for ondansetron than for metoclopramide (£47.60 versus £20.28). The cost per successfully treated patient (obtained by dividing the mean overall utilisation cost per patient by the probability of being successfully treated) was £95.20 for ondansetron and £92.18 for metoclopramide. These results suggest that ondansetron is nearly as effective as metoclopramide in this setting. However, the number of patients was small and a sensitivity analysis was not provided. Corticosteroids were allowed if they were part of the chemotherapy regimen or for physiological supplementation, and it is not known if this treatment was balanced in the two groups of patients.

In a second study [38], a pre-marketing economic evaluation combined secondary analysis of data from a large clinical trial [47] with estimates of emesis management costs in a UK hospital setting in order to assess the cost-effectiveness of ondansetron (8 mg i.v. leading dose, followed by 1 mg/hour i.v. for 24 hours) compared with metoclopramide (3 mg/kg i.v. leading dose, followed by 0.5 mg/kg/h for 8 hours) in patients treated with highly emetogenic chemotherapy. Results of the cost analysis (original patient-specific data from the clinical trial were used to construct a probability tree for each treatment group) showed that the two antiemetic regimens would have equivalent treatment costs if ondansetron were priced 2.3 times higher (1.6 to 3.5 using a sensitivity analysis) than the £10.00 acquisition of metoclopramide. The cost-effectiveness analysis showed the same trend. However, in this study therapeutic success was defined as two or fewer emetic episodes during 24 hours. Extended hospitalisation costs were also considered, antiemetic administration costs (alcohol, swabs, needles, etc.) were not. It should be noted that the probability of extended hospitalisation may depend on the availability of hospital beds, the attending physician and other factors, and these costs may vary between institutions [48].

In a cost-benefit study by Tanneberger et al. [27] it was estimated that an ondansetron regimen, using total doses of 24 to 32 mg for the acute prophylaxis of emesis due to highly emetogenic chemotherapy, would increase the cost of chemotherapy cycles by no more than 6%, compared with a regimen using metoclopramide 10 mg/kg i.v. plus lorazepam. By means of the real cost-benefit index, the ondansetron regimen was found to be favourable. A recent study from Italy has also shown that ondansetron is cost-effective when compared to a metoclopramide regimen [64].

Cost of Ondansetron in Combination

Sands et al. [36] carried out a cost-effectiveness evaluation of ondansetron (8 mg i.v., single dose) plus dexamethasone (8 mg i.v., 8-h in two doses) compared to combination therapy with metoclopramide (3 mg/kg i.v. loading dose, followed by 8 mg/kg i.v. over 8 hours), dexamethasone (8 mg i.v.) plus lorazepam (1 to 1.5 mg i.v.). The economic analysis was carried out using the clinical data from two studies. In one study, 13 patients received the ondansetron combination during 31 chemotherapy cycles, the complete remission rate was 93%. In the second study, 54 metoclopramide recipients achieved a complete response of 76% (41/54). The authors concluded that the cost per effective treatment (calculated by dividing the cost of the local hospital-discounted drug by complete response rate) was lower for the ondansetron combination (£16.27) than the metoclopramide regimen (£17.35). As these data were collected from two limited studies, they would require confirmation in a larger, randomised, double-blind clinical trial. In addition, adverse events, nursing time, consumption of disposable items and the cost of "rescue" antiemetics were not included in the analysis.

A cost-effectiveness analysis by Cox [11] based on a decision analytic framework (costs associated with antiemetic regimens, management of vomiting-retching and significant antiemetic-related adverse events were combined with the differential probabilities resulting from the trial) was carried out using data from 70 patients randomised to ondansetron (8 mg i.v. loading dose followed by 8 mg 3 times daily during the 5-day period following chemotherapy) compared with 80 patients randomised to metoclopramide (60 mg i.v. loading dose followed by 20 mg 3 times daily during the 5-day period following chemotherapy) both in combination with dexamethasone. Patients included women with breast cancer receiving their first cyclophosphamide (≥500 mg/m^2) based chemotherapy on day 1. The cost per successfully treated patient (= cost per patient divided by the probability of a patient being successfully treated) was £184.00 for ondansetron and £160.00 for metoclopramide. Based on a study by Dicato [3] showing that ondansetron given orally twice daily was as effective as 3 times daily dosing in patients receiving cyclophosphamide (≥500 mg/m^2), the costs per successfully treated patient for ondansetron (£133.00) were lower than for metoclopramide (£160.00).

Cost of Granisetron

A retrospective cost-effectiveness study has been carried out in 22 Swiss patients being treated for malignant disease and naive to chemotherapy, who received cisplatin (>15 mg/m^2 i.v. daily) or etoposide (120 mg/m^2 daily for 5 consecutive days) as hospital inpatients. The patients were randomised to receive either granisetron 40 μg/kg (with an optional two additional daily doses of 40 μg/kg i.v. upon the emergence of symptoms), or the combination of metoclopramide (3 mg/kg i.v. loading dose days 1-2, with an optional dose reduction to 2 mg/kg i.v. on days 3-5, followed by 3 mg/kg i.v. infused over 8 hours) plus dexamethasone (12 mg i.v. daily) [37]. Drug prices were derived from published prices (Documed, 1991) with 33% discount to obtain hospital prices. A methodological model was used for cost assessment based on assessment of routine practice in oncology clinics in the Geneva area. The study shows that although the acquisition costs of metoclopramide plus dexamethasone

(54.94 SFr) were lower than those of granisetron (80 SFr), the total costs were comparable (metoclopramide plus dexamethasone = 95.77 SFr, granisetron = 97.20 SFr). As metoclopramide plus dexamethasone was less effective as an antiemetic and associated with more adverse events than granisetron, total costs (metoclopramide plus dexamethasone = 118.81 SFr, granisetron = 113.73 SFr), cost-efficacy ratio (efficacy ratio divided by total cost; efficacy ratio = total number of patient days with complete remission divided by the total number of treatment days; complete remission = no vomiting or no or only mild nausea per day; metoclopramide plus dexamethasone = 0.42/118.81 = 1:283; granisetron = 0.67/113.73 = 1:170) and the incremental cost-effectiveness ratio (total costs of granisetron minus total cost of metoclopramide plus dexamethasone, divided by the percentage efficacy of granisetron minus the percentage efficacy of metoclopramide plus dexamethasone = 5.02/25) were in favour of granisetron.

A second study [49] was a retrospective antiemetic cost identification of 12 consecutive patients presenting with anticipatory nausea and vomiting during consecutive chemotherapy cycles with moderate to severe emetogenic potential. The antiemetic regimens used were the classic regimen: diphenhydramine 12.5 mg plus prednisolone 25 mg plus dehydrobenzperidol 1.25 mg i.v. up to tid, or metoclopramide 2 or 3 mg/kg i.v. loading dose, followed by 3 or 4 mg/kg i.v. infused over 8 hours plus dexamethasone 20 mg i.v.; or others (in various combinations) such as midazolam 5 mg i.v., domperidone 10 mg p.o. tid, alizapride 50 mg i.v., metoclopramide 10 mg i.v., haloperidol 2.5 mg i.v., thiethylperazine 6.5 mg i.v., chlorpromazine 25 mg p.o. tid: 5-HT_3 receptor antagonists; granisetron 3 mg i.v. up to tid, ondansetron 8 mg i.v. tid, dolasetron mesilate 10-50 mg i.v. The methodology used was as follows: calculation of costs: a) drug costs: antiemetic drug + prophylactic agents; b) added costs: materials + pharmacy costs + nursing costs; c) direct costs: a + b; d) adverse event/failure of treatment costs: additional drugs + materials + nursing, behavioural therapy, and pharmacy costs; e) total costs: c + d. The results show that the total drug costs of the 12 evaluated patients range from 37.30 to 318.70 SFr (mean SFr 143.05). It is known that the incidence of anticipatory nausea and vomiting is about 24%. However, in patients treated with granisetron recent data have shown that the incidence of anticipatory nausea and vomiting is significantly lower (4.6%) during consecutive chemotherapy cycles. The conclusion was that granisetron used as a first-line antiemetic in new patients scheduled for consecutive chemotherapy cycles may reduce the incidence of anticipatory nausea and vomiting and result in long-term economic savings [1].

Decision-Making Analysis

Jones et al. [50] constructed a treatment model which represents a baseline of efficacy and the costs of treating a cohort of patients with conventional antiemetics. Groups of patients who would be expected to receive the most benefit from 5-HT_3 receptor antagonists were identified and then the effect upon costs of using these compounds in a consecutively larger proportion of selected patients was calculated. On the basis of illustrative costs from Cookridge Hospital in the UK, it was concluded that the new antiemetics can be used in acute emesis with substantial clinical benefit, with an increase of 3% to 10% in the total treatment costs. For delayed emesis these compounds have not yet shown clinical advantage, and the increase in total costs of 12% to 34% is not justifiable.

Antiemetic Innovation and the Costs and Benefits of Outpatient Therapy

In an attempt to reduce hospital-related costs, the delivery of health care has shifted from the inpatient "acute"-care hospital to ambulatory-care setting [16]. Johnson et al. as well as Rubenstein et al. documented a significantly shorter length of stay (LOS) for patients receiving ondansetron for highly or moderately emetogenic chemotherapy [16,51]. In Johnson's prospective study, the overall treatment cost stayed the same. In their study of 612 admissions for patients receiving highly or moderately emetogenic chemotherapy, under diagnosis-related group 410 in the US, hospital costs per admission were higher, net hospital revenue per admission was lower, and resource consumption was greater for those patients who never received ondansetron. This shortening of LOS has not been found in a retrospective analysis in another US hospital and some methodological concerns are present in Johnson's study [52]. Nevertheless, Dexter et al. observed, in modelling the effect of abolishing nausea and vomiting in post-anaesthesia patients, a theoretical reduction in cost. It remains to be seen if the emesis related to chemotherapy may be a confounding factor for the overall evaluation of the length of hospital stay. In other words, the frequency of vomiting may not make a difference in the decision to discharge patients [53] unless the symptoms are severe, as for the 20% of patients known to be refractory to setron + dexamethasone-based antiemetic treatment [54,55]. Finally, intangible cost savings of the setrons, as perceived by the patient, nurse and physician, have not yet been evaluated in the cost studies available. Indeed, it seems beneficial to see a patient awake, vomiting less, engaging in conversation, able to read and especially to drive home earlier. There is no doubt that most patients, nurses and physicians would choose a setron-based antiemetic regimen. However, it remains to be seen how much a health-insured or non-insured person is willing to pay for the cost per emesis episode avoided [48,56].

Future Prospects

A pharmacoeconomic analysis of the randomised studies comparing the antiemetic efficacy of the major 5-HT_3 receptor antagonists will yield information that is important for decision-making [35,65-70]. For instance, there is a French retrospective study [71] which uses data from 2 large clinical trials comparing granisetron and ondansetron in patients receiving single-dose or fractionated moderately emetogenic chemotherapy [35,67]. There is also a French cost-minimisation study comparing the same drugs [72]. Both studies favour granisetron as more cost-effective in sensitivity analysis except when the dose of granisetron (3 mg) remains unchanged and the ondansetron dosage is reduced to a single 8 mg intravenous dose. Subsequently, selected dose-finding studies have suggested to reduce the ondansetron dosage.

Identical drug indications, dosage and schedules which also affect future costs should be submitted to the regulatory agencies for approval. This cannot always be the case, as shown by the widespread licensing of ondansetron at markedly different doses. Nevertheless, physicians, pharmacists, third-party reimbursement agencies and pharmaceutical companies should at least be aware of such information and closely follow new indications as mentioned in case-reports and new studies in the medical literature. An international, networking panel of experts in antiemetic care [3,57] should handle this information and recommend updated treatment guidelines, which should be available with a simple mouse click (locally or through the Internet). The panel should consult lawyers to settle the legal aspects and explicate possible financial conflicts of interest. Such a dynamic management protocol [44] is needed in the 1990s to allow easy suggestion, interaction and use by all those involved (patients, medically-related professions, physicians, pharmaceutical companies, reimbursement and regulatory agencies, etc.) [58].

Unless such conduct is promoted by physicians and the medically-related professions, reimbursement or regulatory agencies will have a necessary role of cost decision when paying bills in a cash-limited situation [51]. Unfortunately this may come down to covert rationing (random denial of treatment based on geography, diagnosis, age or insurance company) [59]. Indeed, as shown by pharmacist-investigators, third-party monitoring is successful in ensuring the quality of therapy, reducing prescription error and reducing the cost of a 5-HT_3-based antiemetic treatment in cancer patients [60-62]. Government regulatory agencies should design international drug registration standards to avoid the current costly (in terms of time and money), nation-based registration process [50].

Conclusions

There is no doubt that the eagerly awaited, efficacious 5-HT_3 receptor antagonists have raised justified cost concerns. In fact cost, an old concern, has taken the forefront of 1990s health care in general. The methodology for economic evaluations should be standardised if it is to be used objectively in medical management decisions throughout the variegated health care system. A networking panel of experts would be of help in defining antiemetic treatment guidelines and areas for further research. We have probably already seen the major benefit of cost consideration in therapeutic innovation through pharmaceutical company competition, which has resulted in a significant decrease in the cost of the available medication [63].

Just as statistics has changed opinions regarding the conduct of research studies, so will clinical economic analyses.

Acknowledgement

Dr. V. Kirchner is a research fellow from the Ligue Genevoise contre le Cancer (Switzerland). He has been sponsored by or has conducted sponsored research for SmithKline Beecham Pharmaceuticals, Glaxo Inc., Sandoz, Merck Darmstadt, Marion Merrell Dow Inc., and Farmitalia.

REFERENCES

1 Aapro MS, Kirchner V, Terrey JP: Is anticipatory nausea and vomiting a thing of the past. Br J Cancer 1994 (69):957-960
2 Gralla RJ: Antiemetic treatment for cancer chemotherapy: problem and progress. Support Care Cancer 1994 (2):275-276
3 Dicato MA: Oral treatment with ondansetron in an outpatient setting. Eur J Cancer 1991 (27):S18-S19
4 Hillman AL, Eisenberg JM, Pauly NV et al: Sounding board: avoiding bias in the conduct and reporting of cost-effectiveness research sponsored by pharmaceutical companies. N Engl J Med 1991 (324):1362-1365
5 Drummond MF and Davis L: Economic analysis alongside clinical trials: revisiting the methodological issues. Inst J Technol Assess Health Care 1991 (7):561-573
6 Farewell to promising goodbuys? (editorial) Lancet 1991 (338):416-417
7 Miller JP: Use of cost-benefit analysis in promotional material. Lancet 1991 (338):823-824.
8 Thimothy A: Report of a conference: cost versus benefit in non-surgical management of patients with cancer. Br Med J 1988 (297):471-472
9 Evans RG and Robinson BC: Surgical day care: measurements of the economic payoff. Can Med Ass J 1980 (123):873-880
10 Clark RA, Kris MG, Gralla JR, et al: Serotonin antagonists demonstrate antiemetic effectiveness without extrapyramidal symptoms: analysis of studies with 3 new agents in 155 patients. Proc Am Soc Clin Oncol 1990 (9):322
11 Cox F: Ondansetron - a cost-effective advance in anti-emetic therapy. In: Glaxo (ed) Ondansetron - Global experience and future potential. Palais des Congrès Internationaux, Lyon, France, 9 November 1992 pp 40-44
12 Cunningham D, Gore M, Davidson N et al: The real costs of emesis - An economic analysis of ondansetron vs metoclopramide in controlling emesis in patients receiving chemotherapy for cancer. Eur J Cancer 1993 (29A):303-306
13 Detsky AS NI: A clinician's guide to cost-effectiveness analysis. Ann Intern Med 1990 (113):147-154
14 Dexter F and Tinker JH: Analysis of strategies to decrease postanesthesia care unit costs. Anesthesiology 1995 (82):94-101
15 Rubenstein EB and Elting LS: Re-examination of clinical aspects of pharmacoeconomic analysis. Am J Hosp Pharm 1994 (51):2970-2973
16 Rubenstein EB and Elting LS: Pharmacoeconomic analyses: whose perspective counts and costs the most? Am J Hosp Pharm 1994 (51):1564-1569
17 Rubenstein EB, Elting L, Kurtin D, Mikhail O, Swint M: Outcome of antiemetic prophylaxis among outpatients receiving highly emetic chemotherapy (Abstract). Proc Annual Meeting Am Soc Clin Oncol 1994 (13):A1526
18 Rubenstein EB: Costs and benefits of outpatient therapy. Support Care Cancer 1994 (2):307-311
19 Sackett DL and Gent M: Controversy in counting and attributing events in clinical trials. N Engl J Med 1979 (26):1410-1412
20 Sands R, Roberts JT, Marsh M et al: Low dose ondansetron and dexamethasone: a cost effective alternative to high dose metoclopramide/dexamethasone/lorazepam in the prevention of acute cisplatin induced emesis. Clin Oncol 1992 (4):67-68
21 Smith RN: Safety of ondansetron. Eur J Cancer Clin Oncol 1989 (25):547-550
22 Sox HC, Blatt MA, Higgins MC, Marton KI: Cost effectiveness analysis and cost benefit analysis. In: Sox HC, Blatt MA, Higgins MC, Marton KI (eds) Medical Decision Making. Butterworth-Heinemann, Stonehamm, MA 1988 pp 317-335
23 Stanley A: Meeting report. Delivering the benefits of anti-emetic innovation. Vol 4. Meribel, France 1993
24 Stoddart GL and Drummond MF: How to read clinical journals: VII. To understand an economic evaluation (part A). Can Med Assoc J 1984 (130):1428-1434
25 Stoddart GL and Drummond MF: How to read clinical journals: VII. To understand an economic evaluation (part B). Can Med Assoc J 1984 (130):1542-1549
26 Eisenberg JM, Glick H, Koffer H: Pharmacoeconomics: economic evaluation of pharmaceuticals. In: Strom BL (ed) Pharmacoepidemiology. Churchill Livingstone 1990 pp 325-350
27 Tanneberger ST, Lelli G, Martoni A et al: The antiemetic efficacy and the cost-benefit ratio of ondansetron calculated with a new approach of health technology assessment (real cost-benefit index). J Chemother 1992 (4):326-331

28 Tigh M and Goodman S: Carboplatin versus cisplatin. Lancet 1988 (ii):1372-1373
29 Udvarhelyi IS, Colditz GA, Rai A et al: Cost-effectiveness and cost-benefit analyses in the medical literature: are the methods being used correctly. Ann Intern Med 1992 (116):238-244
30 Warr D, McKinney S, Tannock I: Influence of measurement error on assessment of response to anticancer chemotherapy: proposal for new criteria of tumor response. J Clin Oncol 1984 (2):1040-1046
31 Weinstein MC and Stason WB: Foundations of cost-effectiveness analysis for health and medical practices. N Engl J Med 1977 (296):716-721
32 Wodinsky H, DeAnglis C, Rusthoven J et al: Reevaluating the cost of outpatient cancer chemotherapy. Can Med Ass J 1987 (137):903-906
33 Yarbro JW: Changing cancer care in the 1990s and the cost. Cancer 1990 (67):1718-1727
34 Johnson N and Bosanquet N: Cost effectiveness of 5-hydroxytryptamine 3 receptor antagonists: a retrospective comparison of ondansetron and granisetron. Anti-Cancer Drugs 1995 (6):243-249
35 Noble A, Bremer K, Goedhals L: A double-blind, randomised, cross-over comparison of granisetron and ondansetron in 5-day fractionated chemotherapy: assessment of efficacy, safety and patient preference. Eur J Cancer 1994 (8):1083-1088
36 Sands R, Roberts JT, Marsh M et al: Low dose ondansetron and dexamethasone: a cost effective alternative to high dose metoclopramide/dexamethasone/lorazepam in the prevention of acute cisplatin induced emesis. Clin Oncol 1992 (4):67-68
37 Kirchner V, Aapro M, Alberto P et al: The cost-effectiveness of granisetron compared with metoclopramide plus dexamethasone. Proc Am Soc Clin Oncol 1992 (11):379
38 Buxton MJ and O'Brien BJ. Economic evaluation of ondansetron: preliminary analysis using clinical trial data prior to price setting. Br J Cancer 1992 (19 Suppl):S64-67
39 Freund DA and Dittus RS: Principles of pharmacoeconomic analysis of drug therapy. PharmacoEconomics 1992 (1): 20-32
40 Calman K, McVie J, Soukop M et al: Cost of outpatient chemotherapy. Br J Med 1978 (1):493-494
41 Goodwin P, Feld R, Ward P et al: The cost of cancer therapy. Eur J Cancer 1990 (26):223-225
42 Jenett B and Buxton M: When is treatment for cancer economically justified? J Roy Soc Med 1990 (83):25-28
43 Miles D, Richards M, Reubens R: Cost-effectiveness of cancer chemotherapy. Cancer Topics 1990 (7):141-142
44 Rees G: Cost-effectiveness in oncology. Lancet 1985 (ii):1405-1428
45 Goddard M: The real costs of emesis. Eur J Cancer 1993 (29A):297-298
46 O'Brien BJ, Rusthoven J, Rocchi A et al: Impact of chemotherapy-associated nausea and vomiting on patients' functional status and on costs: survey of five Canadian centres. Can Med Assoc J 1993 (149):296-302
47 Marty M, Pouillart P, School S et al: Comparison of the 5-hydroxytryptamine (serotonin) antagonist ondansetron (GR38032F) with high-dose metoclopramide in the control of cisplatin-induced emesis. N Engl J Med 1990 (322):816-821
48 Plosker GL and Richard JM: Ondansetron: a pharmacoeconomic and quality-of-life evaluation of its antiemetic activity in patients receiving cancer chemotherapy. PharmacoEconomics 1992 (2):285-304
49 Kirchner V, Aapro M, Terrey JP: Antiemetic treatment costs in chemotherapy: the economic evaluation of granisetron. ESMO XVII, Palais des Congrès Internationaux, Lyon, France 1992
50 Jones AL, Lee GJ, Bosanquet N: The budgetary impact of 5-HT_3 receptor antagonists in the management of chemotherapy-induced emesis. Eur J Cancer 1992 (29A):51-56
51 Johnson NE, Nash DB, Carpenter CE et al: Ondansetron: costs and resource utilization in a US teaching hospital setting. PharmacoEconomics 1993 (3): 471-481
52 Foltyn Smith C and Amen RJ: Comparison of seven methods of preparing and administering small-volume injections. Am J Hosp Pharm 1988 (45): 1896-1901
53 Wilder-Smith OH and Borgeat A: Etomidate vs propofol for suspension laryngoscopies. Eur J Anaesthesiol 1991 (8):509
54 Parker SE and Davey PG: Pharmacoeconomics of intravenous drug administration. PharmacoEconomics 1992 (1):103-115
55 Borgeat A: Effects of Diprivan on nausea and vomiting. Ann Fr Anesth Reanim 1994 (13):576-578
56 Peto R, Pike MC, Armitage P et al: Design and analysis of randomized clinical trials requiring prolonged observation of each patient. I. Introduction and design. Br J Cancer 1976 (34):585-612
57 Glatstein E and Makuch RW: Illusion and reality: practical pitfalls in interpreting clinical trials. J Clin Oncol 1984 (2):488-497
58 Rubenstein EB, Hauser AR, Rodriguez MA et al: Phase I-II trials of patient-controlled antiemetic therapy in cancer patients (Abstract). Proc Annual Meeting Am Soc Clin Oncol 1992 (11):A1378
59 Redelmeier DA and Tversky A: Discrepancy between medical decisions for individual patients and for groups. N Engl J Med 1990 (322):1162-1164
60 Ried DL, McKenna DA, Horn JR: Meta-analysis of research on the effect of clinical pharmacokinetics services on therapeutic drug monitoring. Am J Hosp Pharm 1989 (46):945-951
61 Blum KV, Abel SR, Urbanski CJ, Pierce JM: Medication error prevention by pharmacists. Am J Hosp Pharm 1988 (45):1902-1903
62 Dranitsaris G, Warr D, Puodziunas A: A randomized trial of the effects of pharmacist intervention on the cost of antiemetic therapy with ondansetron. Support Care Cancer 1995 (3):183-190
63 Drummond M, Stoddart G, Labelle R et al: Health economics: an introduction for clinicians. Ann Intern Med 1987 (107):88-92
64 Ballatori E, Roila F, Berto P et al: Cost and cost-effectiveness analysis of ondansetron versus metoclopramide regimens. A hospital perspective from Italy. PharmacoEconomics 1994 (5):227-237
65 Navari R, Gandara D, Hesketh P: Comparative clinical trial of granisetron and ondansetron in the pro-

phylaxis of cisplatin-induced emesis. J Clin Oncol 1995 (13):1242-1248
66 Ruff P, Paska W, Goedhals L et al: Ondansetron compared with granisetron in the prophylaxis of cisplatin-induced acute emesis: a multicenter double-blind, randomised, parallel-group study. Oncology 1994 (51):113-118
67 Bonneterre J, Hecquet B et al: Granisetron (iv) compared with ondansetron (iv plus oral) in the prevention of nausea and vomiting induced by moderately emetogenic chemotherapy. A cross-over study. Eur J Cancer Clin Oncol 1996 (in press)
68 Gebbia V, Cannata G, Testa A et al: Ondansetron versus granisetron in the prevention of chemotherapy-induced nausea and vomiting: results of a prospective randomized trial. Cancer 1994 (74): 1945-1952
69 Jantunen I, Muhonen T, Kataja V: 5-HT3 receptor antagonists in the prophylaxis of acute vomiting induced by moderately emetogenic chemotherapy - a randomised study. Eur J Cancer 1993 (12):1669-1672
70 Stewart A, McQuade B, Cronje J et al: Ondansetron compared with granisetron in the prophylaxis of cyclophosphamide-induced emesis in out-patients: a multicentre double-blind, double-dummy, randomised parallel-group. Emesis Study Group for Ondansetron and Granisetron in Breast Cancer Patients. Oncology 1995 (52):202-210
71 Johnson N and Bosanquet N: Cost effectiveness of 5-hydroxytryptamine3 receptor antagonists: a retrospective comparison of ondansetron and granisetron. Anticancer Drugs 1995 (6):243-246
72 Jobet I, Zyguel S, Prugnaud J: Economic evaluation of anti-5HT3: development of an economic model for cost minimisation study. J Pharm Clin 1995 (14): 243-249

Alternative Therapies in the Treatment of Chemotherapy-Induced Nausea and Vomiting

Jørn Herrstedt

Department of Medicine/Medical Oncology F, Hillerød Hospital, Helsevej 2, 3400 Hillerød, Denmark

Although it is generally recognised that unorthodox therapies have no objective antitumour activity [1], it is estimated that 30-50% of cancer patients use these unproven methods either alone or along with established cancer therapies [2,3]. Physicians therefore have to be acquainted with alternative therapies, which will only disappear when the majority of malignancies are cured. A large proportion of patients using alternative therapies do so in an attempt to improve resistance and quality of life by mitigating the side-effects of chemotherapy or radiotherapy [3].

Nausea and vomiting are the most frequent side-effects of cancer chemotherapy and the most difficult to tolerate [4,5]. The 5-HT_3 antagonists have improved the treatment of acute chemotherapy-induced nausea and vomiting, but none of these drugs seem preferable to conventional antiemetics in the treatment of delayed emesis, and only a few studies on patients with anticipatory nausea and vomiting have been initiated. Combinations of a 5-HT_3 antagonist and a steroid [6-8] or a dopamine D_2 antagonist [9] further improve the antiemetic effect, but complete protection is still not obtained in all patients. This justifies the continuing search for alternative approaches in the treatment of emesis.

The effect of acupuncture, alone or in combination with conventional antiemetics, has been investigated against acute chemotherapy-induced emesis only. In contrast, behavioural treatments including hypnosis, progressive muscle relaxation training with or without guided visual imagery, systemic desensitisation, taste blocking and cognitive diversion techniques (music therapy, video games) have primarily been investigated in patients with anticipatory nausea and vomiting. This chapter will review the previously published research into the use of these alternative antiemetic therapies.

Acupuncture

Acupuncture (ACP) was first investigated as a treatment for hyperemesis gravidarum, postoperative emesis [10] and pain [11]. These studies showed ACP to be effective against pain and emesis but also revealed some of the methodological problems in ACP trials. First a short review of the ACP trials in postoperative emesis is given as they constitute the basis for ACP research in chemotherapy-induced nausea and vomiting.

ACP and Postoperative Nausea and Vomiting

ACP is applied by inserting a needle into the P6 point (Neiguan point on the pericardial "meridian", two "cun" (Chinese inches) from the distal wrist crease, between the tendons of the palmaris longus and flexor carpii radialis) and subsequently using manual rotation or electrostimulation. Also acupressure (AP) and transcutaneous electrical nerve stimulation (TENS) have been investigated.

In an open trial including 20 patients undergoing minor gynaecological procedures, the effect of 5 minutes of manual ACP on opioid-induced nausea and vomiting was investigated [12]. Significantly less nausea and vomiting was seen in the first postoperative hour compared with a group of 40 similar patients receiving the opioid alone. In an attempt to conduct a double-blind study, Dundee et al. randomly divided 75 patients into 3 groups receiving needling at a "dummy" point, needling at P6 (ACP) or no needling (controls) as treatment for opioid-induced postoperative nausea and vomiting. ACP patients had significantly less emesis than the controls and no difference was observed between controls and patients receiving needling at the "dummy" point [13]. In a retrospective study the same group [14] found that the best results with ACP were obtained when the patients' dominant forearm was used. The clinical relevance of this was questioned as only 7% of the patients were left-handed.

Three additional problems were studied in postoperative trials: 1) manual versus electrical stimulation, 2) the effect of acupressure, and 3) correct timing of ACP in relation to the emetic stimulus. In a prospective, randomised, open study the antiemetic effect of manual needling for 5 minutes was compared to electrical stimulation and to the effect of the antiemetic cyclizine in women premedicated with nalbuphine 10 mg and scheduled for minor gynaecological operations [15]. The study showed the importance of using the correct electrical frequency, as 1000 Hz for 5 minutes and 10 Hz for 15 minutes both induced nausea and/or vomiting in a large proportion of patients. When electrical stimulation was given at 10 Hz for 5 minutes, no significant difference was seen between ACP (manual needling), cyclizine and electrical stimulation. Taking into account the small sample size (31 patients in each group), the risk of a type 2 error is obvious. In a study by Fry 500 consecutive patients undergoing anaesthesia were randomly assigned to a group receiving acupressure and a control group [16]. In the treatment group patients had acupressure applied to the front of the wrist for 30 seconds just before induction of anaesthesia and for another 30 seconds before leaving the operating theatre. Patients in the control group were given similar anaesthetics for the category of operation, but acupressure was not performed. Eleven patients in the acupressure group and 40 in the control group "felt sick" ($p < 0.001$), but the effect of acupressure was brief, 5-30 min. As only 16% (40/250) in the control group felt sick, the emetic potential of premedication and anaesthetics was low, making it difficult to draw conclusions from this study. In a study by Weightman et al. ACP did not lead to a significant reduction in postoperative nausea and vomiting [17]. To make the study single-blind, ACP was performed during surgery and not given prophylactically as in most studies. It was claimed by others [18] that the timing of ACP in relation to induction of the emetic stimulus (premedication) might be crucial and that ACP should be initiated before the onset of the emetic stimulus.

In a recent randomised trial involving 103 women TENS significantly reduced the incidence of vomiting after hysterectomy [19]. The effect was, however, short-lasting as no difference was seen between women receiving TENS and women in the control group 2 hours after discontinuation of TENS.

ACP and Chemotherapy-Induced Nausea and Vomiting

An overview of studies is given in Table 1. In a randomised study metoclopramide 10 mg i.v. was compared with ACP in 20 patients receiving their first course of moderately emetogenic chemotherapy [20]. Only the first 8 hours after chemotherapy were evaluated and no significant difference was seen. However, the dose of metoclopramide used seems insufficient as other trials have demonstrated that a 10-20 mg dose of metoclopramide is no better than placebo [21,22]. As to the short (8-hour) period of observation, it is noteworthy that 55% of the patients received cyclophosphamide-based chemotherapy, since nausea and vomiting after cyclophosphamide is delayed 6-12 hours and peak symptoms are seen at 12 hours [23].

Dundee et al. investigated 105 patients with a history of "troublesome nausea and/or vomiting" following previous cancer chemotherapy [24]. The ACP-technique used was electrostimulation with 10 Hz for 5 min. Patients received the same antiemetics (metoclopramide plus prednisolone) as in the previous course of chemotherapy and were asked to grade their sickness on a 4-point scale: A, worse than before; B, same as before; C, less than before; D, completely absent. The effects of ACP were classified as very good (D), good (C) or poor (A+B), and the results are given in Table 2. Ninety-four percent (99/105) of the patients had some benefit of combining ACP with metoclopramide and prednisolone, but the lack

Table 1. Studies on the use of acupuncture (ACP) in the treatment of chemotherapy-induced nausea and vomiting

Study	Patients	Design	ACP technique	Assessment (N and V)	CT and Antiemetics	Results
Saller et al [28] (1986)	22(43-66 Y) pt with ANV not included	Rand, DB AE + TENS vs AE + placebo	TENS 18+12+5 h before CT and continuously from -2 to 24 h after CT	Pt graded N and V on a 4-point scale 24 h after CT	CIS (60-90 mg/m^2) + BLEO or VDS, AE = MCP 3.5 mg/kg/24 h	AE + TENS superior in reducing V and duration + intensity of N
Dundee et al [25] (1987)	10 (age?) with "sickness after CT"	Single subject	Electro-ACP at P6 or at "dummy" point every 8 h	Effect graded (by pt?) every 8 h on a 4-point scale. P6-ACP compared with "dummy" ACP periods	CIS (30 mg) + other AE not specified	ACP at P6 superior to ACP at "dummy" point
Dundee et al [20] (1988)	20 (age?) CT-naive	Rand to MCP vs ACP	Electro-ACP before CT	Severity of symptoms was "graded on a clinical basis" 8-10 h after CT	CT=CIS, CAV, Mit or CMF. AE=MCP 10 mg x 1 i.v.	No significant difference
Dundee et al [24] (1989)	105 (age?) with "troublesome N and/or V after CT"	Single subject	Electro-ACP before CT and repeated if necessary	Sickness graded by pt on a 4-point scale (after 24 h?). Comparison with pt previous experience	CT=CIS, A, CMF, CAV, Mit. AE=MCP+PRED	94% of the pt had some benefit
Dundee et al [26] (1990)	40 (age?) with "troublesome sickness" at previous CT	Single subject	Electro-ACP before CT and followed by acupressure every 2 h for 24 h	Pt graded as above. In-pt after 8 and 24 h. Out-pt were seen 1-3 weeks after	CT not specified AE="standard AE"	95% of in-pt had some benefit, out-pt did worse
Aglietti et al [27] (1990)	26 (36-74 Y) 22 CT-naive	Compared with a group of historical controls (CT-naive, same CT and AE)	Manual ACP during CIS infusion + pt selfadministration during 24 h if they felt nauseated	Pt graded intensity of N on a 4-point scale at 2, 4, 6, 8 and 24 h after CT. RN counted number of V.	CT=CIS 50-120 mg/m^2 + others. AE=MCP+DX+DP (3 mg/kg x 2, 20 mg x 1 and 50 mg x 1, all i.v.)	AE+ACP significantly superior to AE alone in complete protection from N and mean number of V

A=anticipatory, N=nausea, V=vomiting, Pt=patients, RN=registered nurse, CT=chemotherapy, AE=antiemetics, Y=years, Rand=randomised, DB= double blind, CIS=cisplatin, BLEO=bleomycin, VDS=vindesine, MTX=methotrexate, C=cyclophosphamide, A=adriamycin, V=vincristine, F=5-FU, Mit=mitozantrone, MCP=metoclopramide, PRED=prednisolone, DX=dexamethasone, DP=diphenhydramine
TENS= transcutaneous electrical nerve stimulation

Table 2. Effects of P6 electroacupuncture in 105 patients who were sick following a previous course of cancer chemotherapy

				BENEFIT		
No.	**Sex**	**Malignancy**	**CT**	**Very good**	**Good**	**Poor**
Inpatients						
29	Ma	Testes	Cis+E+B	16	12	1
5	Fe	Lymphoma	C+D+V+/-P	2	3	0
Outpatients						
28	Fe	Breast	Mit	19	9	0
36	Fe	Breast	C+M+F	27	6	3
7	Ma/Fe	Lymphoma	C+D+V+/-P	2	3	2

Ma = male, Fe = female, Cis = cisplatin, E = etoposide, B = bleomycin, Mit = mitozantrone, C = cyclophosphamide, M = methotrexate, CT = chemotherapy, F = 5-fluorouracil, D = doxorubicin, V = vincristine, P = prednisolone (from reference 24)

of precise inclusion criteria and of a control group impairs the conclusions. Furthermore, as pointed out by the authors, the emotional expectation-placebo aspect may play an important role in this study.

In a small cross-over study in 10 patients with severe cisplatin-induced emesis despite metoclopramide, P6-ACP showed a short-lasting effect, while ACP at a "dummy point" was ineffective [25]. The brevity of the effect of ACP is also known from studies on postoperative emesis. Patients often require repeat ACP on the evening of their treatment which necessitates a home or hospital visit, making ACP as described here too time-consuming to be adopted as a routine procedure. Therefore acupressure was investigated in an attempt to prolong the antiemetic effect of ACP. One study included 40 patients who had "troublesome sickness" after a previous course of chemotherapy [26]. All received standard antiemetics and electrical ACP on their dominant forearm (10 Hz for 5 min at P6) before chemotherapy. A seaband was applied immediately after ACP and patients were instructed to press the stud for 5 minutes every 2 hours. The authors claimed that acupressure prolonged the antiemetic effect of ACP, though no comparative group receiving antiemetics and ACP only was included. Inpatients seemed to do better than outpatients although the emetogenic potential of the chemotherapy of inpatients was higher. The explanation given by the authors was that inpatients could be encouraged to use the acupressure prophylactically, while many of the outpatients seemed to resort to acupressure only when they felt sick.

Aglietti et al. [27] treated 26 women with manual ACP before they received cisplatin-based chemotherapy. To maintain the antiemetic effect the needle was replaced by a needle for permanent use which was removed after 24 hours. If nausea occurred patients were instructed to press the needle gently until the symptoms subsided. All patients also received metoclopramide, dexamethasone and diphenhydramine. The antiemetic effect was compared to a group of historical controls receiving the same chemotherapy and antiemetic treatment without ACP. Both groups were evaluated according to well-established criteria. No differences between the two groups were seen in complete protection from nausea and vomiting or from vomiting alone, but ACP clearly increased the number of patients with complete protection from nausea, and decreased the median number of vomiting episodes and duration of nausea and vomiting. Again the method was considered too time-consuming to become a standard antiemetic treatment.

Saller et al. examined the effect of transcutaneous electrical nerve stimulation (TENS) on cisplatin-induced emesis [28]. In a double-blind study 22 patients (20 men) receiving cisplatin-based chemotherapy (60-90 mg/m^2) were randomised to metoclopramide (loading dose 0.25

mg/kg/h for 2 hours followed by continuous infusion of 0.125 mg/kg/h for 24 hours) plus TENS or metoclopramide alone. TENS was given as a 1-hour stimulation 18, 12 and 5 hours before the start of cisplatin and was also performed continuously for 26 hours starting 2 hours before cisplatin. A reduction in the number of emetic episodes, the intensity and the duration of nausea was seen in the TENS-group. Although the study was randomised, the small sample size makes it difficult to be sure that risk factors for the development of emesis such as number of previous chemotherapy courses and dose of cisplatin were equally distributed between the two arms. Furthermore, the same group (and other groups) had previously shown that higher doses of metoclopramide than were used in this study are necessary to prevent cisplatin-induced nausea and vomiting [29].

In summary, the effect of ACP, AP and TENS on acute chemotherapy-induced nausea and vomiting has been investigated. It seems important that ACP is initiated before the introduction of the emetic stimulus. This is in concordance with the prophylactic use of antiemetics. All but one [20] of the studies quoted used ACP in addition to antiemetics, and according to Dundee et al. [24], ACP and AP are only adjuvants to standard antiemetic treatment. Most studies report a positive, but short-lasting effect of ACP, making these methods too time-consuming to be adapted for routine use.

Behavioural Techniques

The use of behavioural interventions in cancer patients to control the adverse reactions to chemotherapy has been previously reviewed [30-36]. These techniques have primarily been applied to patients with anticipatory nausea and vomiting (ANV). In retrospective studies numerous factors have been positively correlated with the risk of developing ANV. The most important among these are the number of chemotherapy courses [33], development of postchemotherapy nausea and vomiting [37, 38], age (<50 years) [39,40], and the susceptibility to motion sickness [41,42]. The importance of anxiety is not clear. In several retrospective studies anxiety was positively correlated to the development of ANV. This was supported by a prospective study by Andrykowski et al. [43], but could not be confirmed in a later study by the same group [44].

Several hypotheses have been proposed to explain the development of ANV [34]; the one that is most widely accepted considers ANV to be an associative learning process. An association is established between the nausea and vomiting directly caused by chemotherapy and various stimuli such as the nurse, the chemotherapy unit, smells, tastes etc. Induction of one or more of these associations takes some time and ANV is therefore generally not a major problem during the initial 1-3 courses of chemotherapy. The conditioned response hypothesis was investigated in a randomised study in which 48 chemotherapy-naive women with stage I-II breast cancer who were started on adjuvant chemotherapy, were randomly allocated to an experimental group (exposed to a distinctive stimulus before chemotherapy) or a control group. After repeated infusions of chemotherapy, the experimental group had increased nausea following presentation of the stimulus (in a location not associated with chemotherapy) whereas the control group had not [45]. The use of behavioural techniques in the treatment of ANV from chemotherapy is based on the attempt to prevent or ameliorate these conditioned responses [46].

There is an abundant literature on behavioural techniques, especially hypnosis and progressive muscle relaxation training (PMRT). Multiple case stories were published 10-15 years ago [47-50], and case stories of hypnosis [51, 52] and other behavioural techniques [53,54] are still appearing. Today it is recognised, however, that in order to progress, behavioural studies should use control groups and proper methodology [34]. Most behavioural trials have not been restricted to the evaluation of nausea and vomiting, but have also included evaluation of pain, depression, anxiety etc. In the following only data concerning nausea and vomiting are reviewed.

Hypnosis

Hypnosis is probably still the most used behavioural technique in children. Children differ from adults in that they are more readily hypnotised [55]. They appear to achieve deep trance quickly, but are noticeably slower in awakening than adults. On the other hand, children are often bored with the progressive muscle relaxation technique frequently used in adults [56]. This explains the age difference between patients participating in studies on the use of hypnosis and of progressive muscle relaxation training (Tables 3 and 4).

An overview of "controlled studies" is given in Table 3. It should be noted that the early studies use the patient as his own control (single subject) in comparing consecutive cycles of chemotherapy, whereas the most recent studies are randomised, including a control group. Zeltzer and colleagues studied for many years the use of hypnosis in children and adolescents [57-60]. In their first study 12 adolescents with a variety of malignancies and "problems with nausea and vomiting" were included [57]. The patients graded the number of vomiting episodes on a 1-10 scale and also reported duration, whereas nausea was not assessed. No control group was included, but patients were followed through a baseline session without hypnotic intervention and the results were compared with those obtained after hypnosis. Eight patients were evaluable and had a significant reduction in the number of vomits; 6 of these also reduced the duration of vomits. In a preliminary study [58] 8 adolescents were followed through 2-3 baseline sessions (preintervention) and then compared with 2-3 sessions where behavioural intervention (a combination of relaxation and distraction) was applied. Patients and a parent rated vomiting and nausea (1-10 point scale) 3-5 days after chemotherapy. Again intervention reduced nausea and vomiting. In the third study the group improved their methodology by randomising patients to hypnosis or supportive counselling [59]. Compared with 2 baseline sessions nausea and vomiting were reduced in both groups and the effect was maintained in a follow-up session without hypnosis or counselling. No differences were seen between the groups, but the small sample size (9 randomised to hypnosis and 10 to control) constituted a substantial risk for overlooking a possible difference. In a recent trial [60] Zeltzer et al. included 54 children and adolescents from a larger population of paediatric oncology patients. Only patients who reported significant nausea and/or vomiting (>3 on a 0-10 scale) were included. After a baseline session of chemotherapy, patients were interviewed about ANV and antiemetic use prior to chemotherapy. Twenty-four hours after chemotherapy patients and a parent were interviewed for postchemotherapy symptoms. Before the next cycle of chemotherapy, patients were randomised to hypnosis (21), cognitive distraction/relaxation (16) or control (17) and followed with the same assessment procedures as above. There were no differences between groups according to baseline measurements of emetogenicity of chemotherapy and use of antiemetics. Hypnosis and distraction were significantly superior to control in reducing the duration (but not the severity) of nausea, and hypnosis also in reducing the duration of vomiting. In a study by Cotanch et al. [61], 12 children receiving chemotherapy were randomised to self-hypnosis/relaxation or control. Hypnosis was reported to reduce nausea and vomiting compared with control.

Two studies addressed the use of hypnosis in the treatment of chemotherapy-induced nausea and vomiting in adults (Table 3). In a small study 6 patients were followed during 7-14 baseline sessions of chemotherapy during which they all developed anticipatory vomiting. During the subsequent 3-5 cycles of chemotherapy deep muscle relaxation hypnosis was able to reduce nausea and vomiting in all patients. The period of assessment was, however, restricted to the time of the actual chemotherapy injection [62]. In another study by Syrjala et al. [63] 67 bone marrow transplant patients were randomly assigned to 1 of 4 groups prior to transplantation conditioning: 1) hypnosis training; 2) cognitive behavioural training; 3) therapist contact control; 4) treatment as usual (control). Patients graded nausea on a visual analogue scale and number of vomits on a 0-3 scale daily until 20 days posttransplant. Only 45 patients completed the study, and therefore 12, 11, 12, and 10 patients were evaluable for response. Nausea and emesis did not differ significantly among groups.

Progressive Muscle Relaxation Training (PMRT)

PMRT is the most widely investigated psychological technique in patients receiving chemotherapy [34]. The technique involves learning

Table 3. "Controlled" studies on the use of hypnosis in the treatment of chemotherapy-induced nausea and vomiting

Study	Patients	Design	Protocol	Assessment (N and V)	CT and Antiemetics	Results
Redd et al [62] (1982)	6 (24-56 Y) with AV	Single subject	7-14 BS 3- 5 TS	N by pt on VAS V by RN, prior to and after CT	CMF (4), MOPP (1) MTX+CTX+ADM+ VCR (1), AE not specified	Less N and V during all TS
Zeltzer et al [57] (1983)	12 (10-20 Y) with "N and V problems"	Single subject	1 BS 1 TS	V rated (1-10) by pt prior to CT and again ?	MOPP and related CT, CPZ (5), marijuana (1)	8 pt reduced frequency and 6 duration of V
LeBaron et al [58] (1984)	8 (10-17 Y) with V	Single subject	2- 3 BS 2- 3 TS	N and V rated (1-10) by pt and parent prior to and 3-5 days after CT	CTX, MTX, VCR, ARA-C AE not specified	7 pt reduced N 8 pt reduced V
Zeltzer et al [59] (1984)	19 (6-17 Y) with N and V	Rand, hypnosis vs counseling	2 BS 2 TS 1 FS	Same as above	CTX, MTX, VCR, ARA-C, MOPP, ADM AE not specified	Reduction of N and V in both groups, no difference between groups
Cotanch et al [61] (1985)	12 (9-18 Y) with "troublesome N and V"	Rand, hypnosis vs control	1 TS 2 FS	N and V by pt on VAS, N and V by RN prior to and 24 h after CT	Not specified	Hypnosis reduced N and V compared with control
Zeltzer et al [60] (1991)	54 (5-17 Y) with N and V more than 3 on a 10 point scale	Rand, hypnosis vs cognitive distraction vs control	1 BS 1 TS	By interview of pt (ANV just after CT) and pt plus parent (post-CT N and V 24 h after CT)	CTX, MTX, ARA-C, DTIC, CIS, AE not specified but "constant during the study"	Duration (not severity) of N and V reduced by hypnosis, duration of N also by distraction.
Syrjala et al [63] (1992)	45 (19-49 Y) undergoing BMT	Rand, hypnosis vs cognitive behavioral training vs therapist control vs control	1 TS	N by pt on VAS, V graded by pt as 0-3 daily for 20 days	Not specified	No significant differences between groups in N and V

A=anticipatory, N=nausea, V=vomiting, BS=baseline sessions, TS=treatment sessions, FS=follow up sessions, Pt=patients, RN=registered nurse, VAS=visual analogue scale, CT=chemotherapy, AE=antiemetics, Y=years, Rand=randomised, BMT=bone marrow transplantation, MOPP=prednisone + procarbazine + nitrogen mustard + vincristine, DTIC=dacarbazine, CIS=cisplatin, MTX=methotrexate, CTX=cyclophosphamide, ADM=adriamycin, VCR=vincristine, CMF=CTX +MTX + 5-FU, ARA-C=cytosine arabinoside, CPZ=chlorpromazine

how to relax by actively tensing and relaxing muscle groups in a progressive manner [33]. Often the patient is taught PMRT by a therapist and a training audiotape is made for practice at home. PMRT is usually combined with guided imagery (GI) individualised to each patient based on preintervention interviews [34]. As with hypnosis the research on PMRT has been dominated by a single group (Table 4). Burish et al. started their research by reporting a case story [49], but soon progressed to randomised studies [64-67]. Initially they randomised 16 patients with anticipatory nausea or vomiting to PMRT plus GI or control. Both groups received "standard antiemetics", graded nausea before and after chemotherapy and were followed for 5 consecutive cycles of chemotherapy. The initial course was a baseline session (BS) with no interventions except for antiemetics. This was followed by two training sessions (TS) and finally by two follow-up sessions (FS). They found significantly less nausea in the PMRT plus GI group, an effect that was preserved during FS. As only two patients in each group vomited during TS and FS, no difference in vomiting was present. So far, PMRT studies had only focused on the time shortly before and during chemotherapy. To investigate if the effect of behavioural intervention was extended beyond this period, in their next study the group prolonged the observation period to 36 hours after chemotherapy (Table 4). It was also recognised that the success of PMRT could be due to therapists' attention and support accompanying PMRT, and therefore the study randomised patients to PMRT plus GI, control (antiemetics only) or therapist control. Patients in the therapist control group received therapists' attention and support, but relaxation was not provided [65]. PMRT plus GI significantly reduced nausea during chemotherapy and during the following 36 hours whereas no difference in vomiting was seen. Having shown that the effect of PMRT was not due to therapists' attention and support and not limited to the period just before and after chemotherapy, Burish et al. randomised 24 chemotherapy-naive patients to PMRT plus GI or control during 5 cycles of chemotherapy [66]. The study confirmed previous results, but also revealed the effect of PMRT plus GI on conditioned nausea and vomiting as less patients in the experimental group had ANV by the 4th-5th cycle of chemotherapy. One of the drawbacks of behavioural techniques is the cost (time) of providing these treatments and the lack of therapists that master them. Unfortunately a study by Carish and Burish [67] showed that PMRT plus GI given by a professional was superior to PMRT plus GI given by a volunteer or by audiotape (Table 4).

Others have also investigated the effect of PMRT. In a preliminary study by Cotanch [68] on patients with ANV induced by previous chemotherapy, nausea and vomiting was reduced in 9 out of 12 patients. In a randomised study including 60 chemotherapy-naive patients, the effect of PMRT versus relaxing music versus control was investigated. Patients were followed during 4-5 consecutive cycles of chemotherapy (1 BS and 3-4 TS). Vomiting but not nausea was significantly reduced by PMRT [69].

Two studies reported negative results on the effect of PMRT plus GI (Table 4). In all the above-mentioned studies patients received antiemetics with or without PMRT plus GI. The study by Scott et al. [70] is interesting because a direct comparison was made between the effect of antiemetics and of PMRT plus GI (Table 4). Seventeen women with stage II-IV ovarian cancer, receiving their first course of high-dose cisplatin-based chemotherapy, were randomised to PMRT plus GI or antiemetic treatment with metoclopramide plus dexamethasone plus diphenhydramine. The number of vomits was significantly reduced by antiemetics (mean 5 versus 16, $p < 0.01$). The number of vomits in the PMRT plus GI group indicates that this treatment is no better than placebo in patients receiving high-dose cisplatin [71]. In a recent study by Holli [72] 67 patients receiving chemotherapy were randomised to antiemetics plus PMRT (43) or antiemetics alone (24) on a ratio of 2 to 1 (Table 4). No significant differences in the number or duration of vomits were seen during the first 24 hours after chemotherapy; nausea was not assessed.

Systematic Desensitisation (SD)

SD is the behavioural technique of choice for the treatment of phobic anxiety [73]. Some authors suggest that the development of ANV is a component of a phobic response to chemo-

Table 4. "Controlled" studies on the use of progressive muscle relaxation training (PMRT) in the treatment of chemotherapy-induced nausea and vomiting

Study	Patients	Design	Protocol	Assessment (N and V)	CT and Antiemetics	Results
Burish et al [64] (1981)	16 (age ?) with AN or AV	Rand, PMRT+GI vs control	1 BS 2 TS 2 FS	N by pt, N and V by RN on a 7-point scale prior to and after CT	Not specified, but AE "constant during the study"	Less N in the PMRT + GI group. No difference in V
Lyles et al [65] (1982)	50 (age ?) with AN and/or AV	Rand, PMRT+GI vs therapy control vs control	1 BS 3 TS 1 FS	As above, pt also rated N and V during the first 36 h after CT	MOPP, CMF, CIS, AE not specified but "constant" during the study"	Less N during CT and at home in the PMRT + GI group. No difference in V
Cotanch et al [68] (1983)	12 (17-49 Y) with $\geq$ 2 h of N and $\geq$ 10 V after CT	Single subject	1 BS 2-6 TS	N by pt, N and V by RN on a 4-point scale during CT, N and V by pt during the first 48 h after CT	Not specified	N and V "improved" in 9 of 12 pt
Scott et al [70] (1986)	17 (33-75 Y) CT-naive	Rand, PMRT+GI vs antiemetics	1 TS	N and V by RN on a 5-point scale during the first 24 h after CT	CIS (120 mg/m^2)+ADM+ CTX, AE = MCP+DEX+ DPH, the PMRT+GI pt received no AE	No significant difference in N Less V (mean 5 vs 16) in the AE group
Cotanch et al [69] (1987)	60 (17-68 Y) CT-naive	Rand, PMRT vs music vs control	1 BS 3-4 TS	N and V by pt on a 4-point scale during the first 48 h after CT	CT not specified, all pt offered "standard AE"	PMRT + GI significantly reduced V but not N compared with controls
Burish et al [66] (1987)	24 (age ?) CT-naive	Rand, PMRT+GI control	5 TS	N by pt, N and V by RN during CT, N and V by pt 72 h after CT (7-point scale)	CT and AE not specified, "emetogenicity of CT did not differ between groups"	Significantly less N during CT and the following 72 h and no ANV in the PMRT + GI group
Carey et al [67] (1987)	45 (25-73 Y) witn AN	Rand, PMRT+GI by a professional vs by a volunteer vs by audiotape vs control	1 BS 3 TS 1 FS	As above, but pt also did pretreatment ratings	As above	Overall pt trained in PMRT + GI by a professional experienced less distress, but no significant differences in N and V
Holli et al [72] 1993)	67 (19-84 Y) N and V ?	Rand, PMRT vs controls	1 TS	Pt and observer rated V (24 h observation?) N was not assessed	CT not specified, AE = MCP+DEX+LOR (both groups)	No significant difference in V

A=anticipatory, N=nausea, V=vomiting, BS=baseline sessions, TS=treatment sessions, FS=follow up sessions, Pt=patients, RN=registered nurse, CT=chemotherapy, MCP=metoclopramide, DEX=dexamethasone, DPH=diphenhydramine, LOR=lorazepam, GI=guided imagery, AE=antiemetics, Y=years, Rand=randomised, MOPP=prednisone + procarbazine + nitrogen mustard + vincristine, ADM=adriamycin, CMF=CTX + MTX + 5-FU, CIS=cisplatin

therapy [74], and SD has been compared with other behavioural techniques in controlled trials as treatment for ANV. The patient is taught progressive muscle relaxation as a competing response to the maladaptive response of ANV [33]. Then the patient is gradually exposed to a hierarchy of events related to chemotherapy. The treatment stimuli then become associated with relaxation instead of nausea and vomiting. A few case stories have been published [75, 76], but the controlled studies come from a single centre [77,78].

In a study by Morrow et al. [77] 60 patients were randomised to SD (20), counselling (20) or no treatment (20). All patients were about to receive their fourth cycle of chemotherapy and all had ANV. Thirty-seven patients received standard antiemetic medication (e.g. prochlorperazine). Chemotherapy (including doses) was not specified, but there was no difference between groups in tumour type, age and sex. Patients were studied during 4 consecutive cycles of chemotherapy; 2 baseline sessions (without behavioural intervention) were held before randomisation, then behavioural treatment was given and patients were assessed for 2 follow-up sessions. Significantly fewer patients in the SD group reported ANV compared to counselled patients ($p < 0.05$) and untreated patients ($p < 0.01$). In patients who continued to have ANV, severity and duration was reduced by SD.

In another study the effectiveness of SD was compared to PMRT, counselling and no treatment [78]. The study included 92 patients, 60 of whom were primarily entered into the study mentioned above [77]. An additional 20 patients were then assigned to PMRT and finally 12 patients were randomised to SD or PMRT. Again all patients had ANV and were included before the fourth cycle of chemotherapy. Methodology and evaluation was as above, except that vomiting was not assessed. Relative to the other groups, SD patients reported a significant reduction in the severity and duration of anticipatory nausea from baseline to follow-up, but both SD and PMRT reduced posttreatment nausea compared to counselling and no treatment. It was quoted by Morrow and others [34] that due to differences in relaxation techniques (GI was not given and relaxation was not provided during chemotherapy treatments) this study should not be considered as a direct comparison between SD and PMRT.

Other Behavioural Techniques

The use of biofeedback combined with PMRT and GI has been studied in a case report and in a small randomised trial [48,79]. Shartner et al. [79] randomised 12 patients to electromyograph biofeedback plus PMRT or thermal biofeedback plus PMRT or control. Patients were studied during 5 cycles of chemotherapy. The study indicated that biofeedback (both eletromyograph and thermal) combined with PMRT was able to reduce nausea during and after chemotherapy.

The taste of drugs during injections has been suggested to be a predictor of anticipatory nausea [80]. Greene et al. have attempted to mask taste sensations that were thought to function as a conditioned stimulus eliciting anticipatory symptoms. They reported a decrease in anticipatory symptoms with the introduction of the taste masking agent (lemon solution) in a single patient [54]. Another intervention is stress inoculation training, but again very few data are available [81].

It has been suggested that the effect of behavioural interventions might in part be due to the ability of these methods to distract patients' attention from chemotherapy. The study by LeBaron et al. combining cognitive distraction with relaxation [58] has been discussed earlier (Table 4). Others have used music [82,83] or video games [84,85] to distract patients. Redd et al. [85] compared the severity of nausea in 13 children who played video games during chemotherapy with that of a control group who did not. Nausea as assessed on a visual analogue scale was significantly reduced by video games. However, it should be noted that 7 children in the study group but only 3 in the control group received antiemetics. Fifteen children from this initial study participated in a subsequent study. After a no-video-game baseline assessment of 10 minutes, patients played video games for 10 minutes, followed by another 10-minute no-video-game period and finally a second 10-minute video-game period. Again nausea was reduced when patients played video games [85].

In summary, behavioural techniques such as hypnosis, PMRT plus GI and SD have in several trials been effective compared to no treatment. Hypnosis seems preferable in children, whereas PMRT plus GI and SD have been primarily investigated in adults. Other interventions such as biofeedback, stimulus control and cognitive divertion techniques have in a few studies been able to reduce ANV, but data are too limited to allow any conclusions about the utility of these methods. As for ACP, behavioural interventions have almost exclusively been investigated as adjuncts to pharmacological antiemetic treatment. Only one study directly compared the effect of behavioural intervention with antiemetic drug treatment. Antiemetics were significantly superior to hypnosis in reducing the number of vomits in patients receiving highly emetogenic chemotherapy [70]. Recognising the amount of time needed for behavioural intervention techniques, it was investigated if PMRT plus GI could be delivered as effectively by trained paraprofessionals or by audiotape as by experienced psychologists [67]. Unfortunately PMRT plus GI delivered by experienced therapists was superior.

Conclusions

The studies cited in this review suggest that alternative antiemetic treatments such as acupuncture and some behavioural techniques are effective in a number of patients when given as adjuncts to pharmacological antiemetic therapy. Given alone or in patients receiving highly emetogenic chemotherapy, the effect is less pronounced and does not seem to exceed the effect of placebo [63,70]. Unfortunately, most of these therapies are time-consuming and their widespread use is limited by the lack of experts that master them.

Substantial conclusions are impeded by methodological problems. Small sample size and lack of stringent inclusion criteria, resulting in heterogeneous patient populations, are evident problems. Only a few of the studies cited in Tables 1, 3 and 4 include detailed information about combinations and doses of cytostatics, dose reductions of cytostatics during subsequent cycles of chemotherapy and of the antiemetics given. Future studies should optimise the methodology in these aspects. It is noteworthy that assessment criteria have been improved during the last decade. Studies evaluating patients a few hours (just before and during chemotherapy infusion) have been replaced by studies with prolonged follow-up periods. Well-defined assessment scales for nausea and vomiting are often used, but as in conventional antiemetic studies, the need for standard evaluation criteria is obvious. Studies on the use of behavioural interventions have focused primarily on the treatment of ANV. The only drugs with some documented effect on ANV are the benzodiazepines [86,87]. The sedative and amnesic properties of these drugs may be responsible for blockade of the conditioned nausea and vomiting elicited by chemotherapy. This is supported by a study of Razavi et al., in which PMRT combined with the benzodiazepine alprazolam was superior to PMRT alone in delaying the occurrence of anticipatory nausea [88].

The overall prevalence of anticipatory nausea has been estimated to range between 23% and 33%, depending on the number of chemotherapy treatments given [33]. In a recent trial the frequency of anticipatory symptoms was unchanged (33%) but severity was mild [89]. These estimations were done prior to the routine use of the 5-HT_3 receptor antagonists in the treatment of acute chemotherapy-induced nausea and vomiting. Since the best strategy to prevent ANV is aggressive antiemetic treatment during early courses of chemotherapy [90], it is possible that the effectiveness of these drugs on acute emesis might reduce the frequency of ANV. This does not abolish the need for research into alternative antiemetic interventions. With the best pharmacological antiemetic combinations only 60-90% of patients obtain complete protection from emesis during the initial 1-2 courses of cisplatin-based chemotherapy [6-9], and the number of patients with complete protection decreases during subsequent chemotherapy cycles [91]. Furthermore, the inclusion of growth factors and bone marrow transplantation in treatment protocols makes the use of higher doses of chemotherapy possible, thereby increasing the emetogenicity of regimens.

Future research should focus on behavioural techniques as adjuncts to antiemetics in the prophylaxis of ANV. Such a combination might be useful especially in patients where anxiety is an important element [92]. Research should not be restricted to the prevention of nausea, but include other related problems such as chemotherapy-related food aversions [93].

REFERENCES

1 Jallut OB: What can be done against unproven methods in cancer therapy. The Swiss experience. J Cancer Res Clin Oncol 1990 (116, Suppl, Part II):S950

2 Kjær M: Unproven methods in cancer therapy in Denmark and Scandinavia. J Cancer Res Clin Oncol 1990 (116, Suppl, Part II):S949

3 Jungi WF: Alternative medicine (AM) in the German-speaking countries in Europe. J Cancer Res Clin Oncol 1990 (116, Suppl, Part II):S949

4 Coates A, Abraham S, Kaye SB, Sowerbutts T, Frewin C, Fox RM, Tattersall MHN: On the receiving end - patient perception of the side-effects of cancer chemotherapy. Eur J Cancer Clin Oncol 1983 (19):203-208

5 Richardson JL, Marks G, Levine A: The influence of symptoms of disease and side effects of treatment on compliance with cancer therapy. J Clin Oncol 1988 (6):1746-1752

6 Roila F, Tonato M, Cognetti F et al: Prevention of cisplatin-induced emesis: a double-blind multicenter randomized crossover study comparing ondansetron and ondansetron plus dexamethasone. J Clin Oncol 1991 (9):675-678

7 Smyth JF, Coleman RE, Nicolson M et al: Does dexamethasone enhance control of acute cisplatin induced emesis by ondansetron? Br Med J 1991 (303):1423-1426

8 Smith DB, Newlands ES, Rustin GJS et al: Comparison of ondansetron plus dexamethasone as antiemetic prophylaxis during cisplatin-containing chemotherapy. Lancet 1991 (338):487-490

9 Herrstedt J, Sigsgaard T, Boesgaard M, Jensen TP, Dombernowsky: Ondansetron plus metopimazine compared with ondansetron alone in patients receiving moderately emetogenic chemotherapy. N Engl J Med 1993 (328):1076-1080

10 Lewith GT, Lewith NR. Modern Chinese Acupuncture. Thorsons Publishers Ltd, Wellingborough 1980

11 Lewith GT, Machin D: On the evaluation of the clinical effects of acupuncture. Pain 1983 (16):111-127

12 Chestnutt WN, Dundee JW: Acupuncture for relief of meptanozol-induced vomiting. Br J Anaesth 1985 (57):825P-826P

13 Dundee JW, Chestnutt WN, Ghaly RG, Lynas AGA: Traditional Chinese acupuncture: a potentially useful antiemetic? Br Med J 1986 (293):583-584

14 Dundee JW, Fitzpatrick KTJ, Ghaly RG, Patterson CC: Does dextrality or sinistrality affect the outcome of P6 acupuncture anti-emesis? Br J Clin Pharmacol 1988 (25):679P-680P

15 Ghaly RG, Fitzpatrick KTJ, Dundee JW: Antiemetic studies with traditional Chinese acupuncture. A comparison of manual needling with electrical stimulation and commonly used antiemetics. Anaesthesia 1987 (42):1108-1110

16 Fry ENS: Acupressure and postoperative vomiting. Anaesthesia 1986 (41):661-662

17 Weightman WM, Zacharias M, Herbison P: Traditional Chinese acupuncture as an antiemetic. Br Med J 1987 (295):1379-1380

18 Dundee JW, Milligan KR: Acupuncture as an antiemetic. Br Med J 1988 (296):135

19 Fassoulaki A, Papilas K, Sarantopoulos C, Zotou M: Transcutaneous electrical nerve stimulation reduces the incidence of vomiting after hysterectomy. Anesth Analg 1993 (76):1012-1014

20 Dundee JW, Ghaly RG, Fitzpatrick KTJ: Randomised comparison of the antiemetic effects of metoclopramide and electroacupuncture in cancer chemotherapy. Br J Clin Pharmacol 1988 (25):678P-679P

21 Moertel CG, Reitemeier RJ: Controlled clinical studies of orally administered antiemetic drugs. Gastroenterology 1969 (57):262-268

22 Morran C, Smith DC, Anderson DA, McArdle CS: Incidence of nausea and vomiting with cytotoxic chemotherapy: a prospective randomised trial of antiemetics. Br Med J 1979 (1):1323-1324

23 Fetting JH, Grochow LB, Folstein MF, Ettinger DS, Colvin M: The course of nausea and vomiting after high-dose cyclophosphamide. Cancer Treat Rep 1982 (66):1487-1493

24 Dundee JW, Ghaly RH, Fitzpatrick KTJ, Abram WP, Lynch GA: Acupuncture prophylaxis of cancer chemotherapy-induced sickness. J Roy Soc Med 1989 (82):268-271

25 Dundee JW, Ghaly RG, Fitzpatrick KTJ, Lynch GA, Abram WP: Acupuncture to prevent cisplatin-associated vomiting. Lancet 1987 (1):1083

26 Dundee JW, Yang J: Prolongation of the antiemetic action of P6 acupuncture by acupressure in patients having cancer chemotherapy. J Roy Soc Med 1990 (83):360-362

27 Aglietti L, Roila F, Tonato M et al: A pilot study of metoclopramide, dexamethasone, diphenhydramine and acupuncture in women treated with cisplatin. Cancer Chemother Pharmacol 1990 (26):239-240

28 Saller R, Hellenbrecht D, Bühring M, Hess H: Enhancement of the antiemetic action of metoclopramide against cisplatin-induced emesis by transdermal electrical nerve stimulation. J Clin Pharmacol 1986 (26):115-119

29 Saller R, Hellenbrecht D, Hellstern A, Hess H: Improved benefit/risk ratio of higher-dose metoclopramide therapy during cisplatin-induced emesis. Eur J Clin Pharmacol 1985 (29):311-312

30 Redd WH, Andrykowski MA: Behavioral intervention in cancer treatment: controlling aversion reactions to chemotherapy. J Consult Clin Psychol 1982 (50):1018-1029

31 Cotanch PH: Relaxation techniques as antiemetic therapy. In: Laszlo J (ed) Antiemetic and Cancer Chemotherapy. Williams & Wilkins, Baltimore/London 1983 pp 164-176

32 Pratt A, Lazar RM, Penman D, Holland JC: Psychological parameters of chemotherapy-induced conditioned nausea and vomiting: a review. Cancer Nurs 1984 (Dec):483-490

33 Morrow GR, Dobkin PL: Anticipatory nausea and vomiting in cancer patients undergoing chemotherapy treatment: prevalence, etiology, and behavioral interventions. Clin Psychol Rev 1988 (8):517-556

34 Carey MP, Burish TG: Etiology and treatment of the psychological side effects associated with cancer

chemotherapy: a critical review and discussion. Psychol Bulletin 1988 (104):307-325
35 Redd WH, Silberfarb PM, Andersen BL et al: Physiologic and psychobehavioral research in oncology. Cancer 1991 (67):813-822
36 Trijsburg RW, Van Knippenberg FCE: Effects of psychological treatment on cancer patients: a critical review. Psychosomatic Medicine 1992 (54):489-517
37 Wilcox PM, Fetting JH, Nettesheim KM, Abeloff MD: Anticipatory vomiting in women receiving cyclophosphamide, methotrexate, and 5-FU (CMF), adjuvant chemotherapy for breast carcinoma. Cancer Treat Rep 1982 (66):1601-1604
38 Morrow GR: Prevalence and correlates of anticipatory nausea and vomiting during chemotherapy. JNCI 1982 (68):585-588
39 Cohen RE, Blanchard EB, Ruckdeschel JC, Smolen RC: Prevalence and correlates of posttreatment and anticipatory nausea and vomiting in cancer chemotherapy. J Psychosomatic Res 1986 (30): 643-654
40 Fetting JH, Wilcox PM, Iwata BA et al: Anticipatory nausea and vomiting in an ambulatory medical oncology population. Cancer Treat Rep 1983 (67): 1093-1098
41 Leventhal H, Easterling DV, Nerenz DR, Love RR: The role of motion sickness in predicting anticipatory nausea. J Behav Med 1988 (11):117-130
42 Morrow GR: Susceptibility to motion sickness and the development of anticipatory nausea and vomiting in cancer patients. Cancer Treat Rep 1984 (68):99-100
43 Andrykowski MA, Redd WH: Development of anticipatory nausea: a prospective analysis. J Consult Clin Psychol 1985 (53):447-454
44 Andrykowski MA, Jacobsen PB, Marks E et al: Prevalence, predictors, and course of anticipatory nausea in women receiving adjuvant chemotherapy for breast cancer. Cancer 1988 (62):2607-2613
45 Bovbjerg DH, Redd WH, Jacobson PB et al: An experimental analysis of classically conditioned nausea during cancer chemotherapy. Psychosomatic Med 1992 (54):623-637
46 Burish TG, Carey MP: Conditioned aversive responses in cancer chemotherapy patients: theoretical and developmental analysis. J Consult Clin Psychol 1986 (54):593-600
47 Dahlquist LM, Gil KM, Armstrong FD, Ginsberg FD, Jones B: Behavioral management of children's distress during chemotherapy. J Behav Ther Exp Psychiatry 1985 (16):325-329
48 Burish TG, Shartner CD, Lyles JN: Effectiveness of multiple-site EMG biofeedback and relaxation in reducing the aversiveness of cancer chemotherapy. Biofeedback and Selfregulation 1981 (6):523-535
49 Burish TG, Lyles JN: Effectiveness of relaxation training in reducing the aversiveness of chemotherapy in the treatment of cancer. J Behav Ther Exp Psychiatry 1979 (10):357-361
50 Dempster CR, Balson P, Whalen BT: Supportive hypnotherapy during the radical treatment of malignancies. Int J Clin Exp Hypnosis 1976 (24):1-9
51 LaClave LJ, Blix S: Hypnosis in the management of symptoms in a young girl with malignant astrocytoma: a challenge to the therapist. Int J Clin Exp Hypnosis 1989 (37):6-14
52 Kaye JM: Use of hypnosis in the treatment of cancer patients. J Psychosoc Oncology 1987 (5): 11-22
53 Booraem CD, Flowers JV, Gumbiner J: Combined medical and psychological treatment of postchemotherapy nausea and vomiting: a case study. Psychological Rep 1989 (65):187-193
54 Greene PG, Seime RJ: Stimulus control of anticipatory nausea in cancer chemotherapy. J Behav Ther Exp Psychiatry 1987 (18):61-64
55 Olness K: Imagery (self-hypnosis) as adjunct therapy in childhood cancer. Am J Pediatric Hematology/Oncology 1981 (3):313-321
56 Hockenberry MJ, Cotanch PH: Hypnosis as adjuvant antiemetic therapy in childhood cancer. Nurs Clin North Am 1985 (20):105-107
57 Zeltzer L, Kellerman J, Ellenberg L, Dash J: Hypnosis for reduction of vomiting associated with chemotherapy and disease in adolescents with cancer. J Adolescent Health Care 1983 (4):77-84
58 LeBaron S, Zeltzer L: Behavioral intervention for reducing chemotherapy-related nausea and vomiting in adolescents with cancer. J Adolescent Health Care 1984 (5):178-182
59 Zeltzer L, LeBaron S, Zeltzer PM: The effectiveness of behavioral intervention for reduction of nausea and vomiting in children and adolescents receiving chemotherapy. J Clin Oncol 1984 (2):683-690
60 Zeltzer L, Dolgin MJ, LeBaron S, LeBaron C: A randomised, controlled study of behavioral intervention for chemotherapy distress in children with cancer. Pediatrics 1991 (88):34-42
61 Cotanch P, Hockenberry M, Herman S: Self-hypnosis as an antiemetic therapy in children receiving chemotherapy. Oncol Nurs Forum 1985 (12):41-46.
62 Redd WH, Andresen GV, Minagawa RY: Hypnotic control of anticipatory emesis in patients receiving cancer chemotherapy. J Consult Clin Psychology 1982 (50):14-19
63 Syrjala KL, Cummings C, Donaldson GW: Hypnosis or cognitive behavioral training for reduction of pain and nausea during cancer treatment: a controlled clinical trial. Pain 1992 (48):137-146
64 Burish TG, Lyles JN: Effectiveness of relaxation training in reducing adverse reactions to cancer chemotherapy. J Behav Med 1981 (4):65-78
65 Lyles JN, Burish TG, Krozely MG, Oldham RK: Efficacy of relaxation training and guided imagery in reducing the aversiveness of cancer chemotherapy. J Consult Clin Psychology 1982 (50):509-524
66 Burish TG, Carey MP, Krozely MG, Greco FA: Conditioned side effects induced by cancer chemotherapy: prevention through behavioral treatment. J Consult Clin Psychology 1987 (55):42-48
67 Carey MP, Burish TG: Providing relaxation training to cancer chemotherapy patients: a comparison of three delivery techniques. J Consult Clin Psychology 1987 (55): 732-737
68 Cotanch PH: Relaxation training for control of nausea and vomiting in patients receiving chemotherapy. Cancer Nurs 1983 (6):277-283
69 Cotanch PH, Strum S: Progressive muscle relax-

ation as antiemetic therapy for cancer patients. Oncol Nurs Forum 1987 (14):33-37

70 Scott DW, Donahue DC, Mastrovito RC, Hakes TB: Comparative trial of clinical relaxation and an antiemetic drug regimen in reducing chemotherapy-related nausea and vomiting. Cancer Nurs 1986 (9):178-187

71 Gralla RJ, Itri LM, Pisko SE et al: Antiemetic efficacy of high-dose metoclopramide: randomized trials with placebo and prochlorperazine in patients with chemotherapy-induced nausea and vomiting. N Engl J Med 1981 (305):905-909

72 Holli K: Ineffectiveness of relaxation on vomiting induced by cancer chemotherapy. Eur J Cancer 1993 (29A):1915-1916

73 Wolpe J: The Practice of Behavior Therapy (3rd ed). Pergamon Press, Oxford 1983

74 Reesal RT, Bajramovic H, Mai F: Anticipatory nausea and vomiting: a form of chemotherapy phobia? Can J Psychiatry 1990 (35):80-82

75 Hailey BJ, White JG: Systematic desensitization for anticipatory nausea associated with chemotherapy. Psychosomatic 1983 (24):289-291

76 Hoffman ML: Hypnotic desensitization for the management of anticipatory emesis in chemotherapy. Am J Clin Hypnosis 1982-1983 (25):173-176

77 Morrow GR, Morrell C: Behavioral treatment for the anticipatory nausea and vomiting induced by cancer chemotherapy. N Engl J Med 1982 (307):1476-1480

78 Morrow GR: Effect of the cognitive hierarchy in the systematic desensitization treatment of anticipatory nausea in cancer patients: a component comparison with relaxation only, counseling, and no treatment. Cogn Ther Res 1986 (10):421-446

79 Shartner CD, Burish TG, Carey MP: Effectiveness of biofeedback with progressive muscle relaxation training in reducing the aversiveness of cancer chemotherapy: a preliminary report. Jap J Biofeedback Res 1985 (12):33-40

80 Nerenz DR, Leventhal H, Easterling DV, Love RR: Anxiety and taste as predictors of anticipatory nausea in cancer chemotherapy. J Clin Oncol 1986 (4):224-233

81 Moore K, Altmaier EM: Stress inoculation training with cancer patients. Cancer Nurs 1981 (Oct):389-393

82 Frank JM: The effects of music therapy and guided visual imagery on chemotherapy induced nausea and vomiting. Oncology Nursing Forum 1985 (12):47-52

83 Porchet-Munro S: Music therapy in support of cancer patients. In: Senn HJ, Glaus A, Schmid L (eds) Recent Results in Cancer Research: Supportive Care in Cancer Patients. Springer-Verlag, Berlin 1988 pp 289-294

84 Kolko DJ, Rickard-Figueroa JL: Effects of video games on the adverse corollaries of chemotherapy in pediatric oncology patients: a single-case analysis. J Consult Clin Psychology 1985 (53):223-228

85 Redd WH, Jacobsen PB, Die-Trill M et al: Cognitive/attentional distraction in the control of conditioned nausea in pediatric cancer patients receiving chemotherapy. J Consult Clin Psychology 1987 (55):391-395

86 Friedlander M, Kearsley JH, Tattersall MHN: Oral lorazepam to improve tolerance of cytotoxic therapy. Lancet 1981 (1):1316-1317

87 Bishop JF, Olver IN, Wolf MM et al.: Lorazepam: a randomized, double-blind, crossover study of a new antiemetic in patients receiving cytotoxic chemotherapy and prochlorperazine. J Clin Oncol 1984 (2):691-695

88 Razavi D, Delvaux N, Farvacques C et al.: Prevention of adjustment disorders and anticipatory nausea secondary to adjuvant chemotherapy: a double-blind, placebo-controlled study assessing the usefulness of alprazolam. J Clin Oncol 1993 (11):1384-1390

89 Stefanik ME, Sheidler VR, Fetting JH: Anticipatory nausea and vomiting: does it remain a significant problem? Cancer 1988 (62):2654-2657

90 Grunberg SM, Hesketh PJ: Control of chemotherapy-induced emesis. N Engl J Med 1993 (329):1790-1796)

91 Soukop M, McQuade B, Hunter E et al.: Ondansetron compared with metoclopramide in the control of emesis and quality of life during repeated chemotherapy for breast cancer. Oncology 1992 (49):295-304

92 Watson M: Anticipatory nausea and vomiting: broadening the scope of psychological treatments. Support Care Cancer 1993 (1):171-177

93 Redd WH: Advances in behavioural intervention in comprehensive cancer treatment. Support Care Cancer 1994 (2):111-115

Unsolved Problems and Future Prospects

Albano Del Favero [1], Enzo Ballatori [2] and Fausto Roila [3]

1 Institute of Internal Medicine and Oncological Sciences, Policlinico Monteluce, Via Brunamonti, 06122 Perugia
2 Medical Statistics Unit, Department of Internal Medicine and Public Health, University of L'Aquila
3 Medical Oncology Division, Policlinico Monteluce, Via Brunamonti, 06122 Perugia, Italy

Although in the last few years the control of chemotherapy-induced nausea and vomiting has received increasing attention and new antiemetic drugs have been made available, the control of these symptoms is still far from being completely satisfactory.

The unsolved problems can be seen from various perspectives: according to the symptoms (nausea/vomiting; acute/delayed), the type of control (prevention/rescue treatment), the type of chemotherapy (highly/moderately emetogenic) or the type of antiemetic drug/ combination of drugs/schedule used. In all these areas there are several unsolved problems which require consideration and the oncologist is confronted with many of them at the same time.

The aim of this review is to call attention to these unsolved problems in order to stimulate further research into these topics.

Unsolved Problems

For practical purposes we will discuss in separate paragraphs first the problems related to high-dose cisplatin-induced nausea and vomiting, then we will review those concerning the moderately emetogenic chemotherapy.

Highly Emetogenic Chemotherapy

Five main problems can be identified in this area:

1) the unsatisfactory control of acute emesis in some subgroups of patients;
2) the unsatisfactory control of delayed emesis;
3) the identification of the best rescue treatment in patients who fail on usual antiemetic treatment;
4) the decreasing efficacy of antiemetic treatment in subsequent cycles of chemotherapy;
5) the identification of optimal drug combination and/or dose-schedule of administration of available treatments.

These problems concern two groups of patients: those treated with high-dose cisplatin and those receiving "high-dose chemotherapy", including cyclophosphamide and melphalan during autologous bone marrow transplantation procedures. Most of the data on this topic comes from studies on high-dose cisplatin treatment and therefore we will refer mainly to that experience.

The Unsatisfactory Control of Acute Emesis

Results from many randomised controlled studies indicate that despite the good overall complete protection (60-80% of patients) achieved with the combination of a 5-HT_3 antagonist with steroid, some patients such as young subjects, females, and patients with previous experience of nausea and/or vomiting induced by chemotherapy, are not protected in the same satisfactory way [1]. An improvement in complete protection from acute emesis can come from new drugs or a combination of drugs.

Is there any chance that a new 5-HT_3 antagonist has greater efficacy than the other compounds?

Animal experiments [2] indicated possible differences among 5-HT_3 receptor antagonists on the basis of the following observations:

1. Ondansetron seems to have a weak antagonistic activity on 5-HT_{1B}, 5-HT_{1C} and $\alpha 1$ and μ receptors. This problem has been discussed with contrasting positions: some authors suggest that similar activity is also present with granisetron and tropisetron [3] while others state that these latter 5-HT_3 antagonists seem more selective with respect to 5-HT_3 receptors [4]. In any case, all three drugs have a selectivity ratio of about 1000:1 for the 5-HT_3 receptors with respect to any other type of receptor. Therefore, it is unlikely that the weak antagonistic activity on other receptors has clinical relevance.
2. The duration of action and the potency of ondansetron is less than that of the other 5-HT_3 antagonists. This does not necessarily mean that repeated doses of ondansetron are required. In fact, at least three studies showed that the single dose works as well as repeated i.v. doses or as a continuous infusion [5-7]. Probably the antiemetic efficacy of 5-HT_3 antagonists is not correlated with their plasmatic level but with the duration and intensity of inhibition of central and peripheral 5-HT_3 receptors.
3. A linear dose-response correlation has been demonstrated with granisetron and tropisetron but not with ondansetron [2]. It seems that in ferrets submitted to cisplatin and receiving ondansetron as an antiemetic, after an initial decrease in emesis at higher doses of ondansetron the protection decreases.
4. Finally, while in the rat there is an insurmountable antagonism of granisetron and tropisetron to 5-HT_3 receptors, in the case of ondansetron the antagonism was overcome by increasing the concentration of 5-hydroxytryptamine.

All these observations stimulated comparative clinical trials among the three available 5-HT_3 antagonists (ondansetron, granisetron, tropisetron).

To date, 10 comparative studies have been published [8-17], 4 in abstract form only [10,11, 13,16]. Four studies [8-11] involved cisplatin-treated patients, 5 [12-16] patients receiving moderately emetogenic chemotherapy and one study involved both types of patients [17]. Unfortunately, these studies have not provided convincing data on possible differences among the 5-HT_3 antagonists. This is because, independent of the contrasting results reported, these trials have some important shortcomings such as: the patient population studied was generally not large enough to be able to show small but still clinically important differences; the design of 8 of 10 of these studies [10-17] was open to criticism because treatments were not blinded; in all but one study [12] the serotonin receptor antagonist was not used in combination with dexamethasone as it should be done to maximise treatment efficacy [1,18].

At the 1995 American Society of Clinical Oncology meeting three large, well conducted comparative trials among 5-HT_3 antagonists were presented (Table 1). Two of these trials were sponsored by pharmaceutical industries and did not associate corticosteroids with the 5-HT_3 antagonists [19-20]. The results of these studies clearly indicate that clinically important differences (i.e. >10% in terms of complete protection from vomiting) do not exist among the 5-HT_3 receptor antagonists studied, such as ondansetron, the comparative drug in all three studies, granisetron and dolasetron. On the basis of these data it seems unlikely that any new 5-HT_3 compound will provide a real advance in antiemetic treatment with respect to the parent compound already available.

What is the role of the drug combinations?

There is now enough evidence to support the routine use of dexamethasone as an adjuvant to 5-HT_3 antagonists (as well as other antiemetic compounds) for treatment of acute emesis [1,18].

Contrasting results come from the search of other, even more effective drug combinations. In fact, while in a small pilot study the addition of ondansetron to the combination of metoclopramide plus dexamethasone plus lorazepam did not improve vomiting prevention in high-dose cisplatin-treated patients [22], more recently a combination of a 5-HT_3 antagonist and a selective D_2 antagonist has been demonstrated to be superior to the 5-HT_3 antagonist alone. In fact, in 111 patients submitted to cisplatin, 70-100 mg/m^2 ondansetron plus meto-

Table 1. Double-blind randomised trials among the 5-HT_3 antagonists in cisplatin-treated patients

No. pts	Dose CDDP (mg/m^2)	Antiemetics	C.P.	Results	Ref.
198		DOL 1.8 mg/kg iv	44.4	1.8 = 2.4 mg/kg DOL = 32mg OND	
205	≥60	DOL 2.4 mg/kg iv	40.0		19
206		OND 32 mg iv	42.7		
328		GRAN 10 μg/kg iv	47	10 μg/kg=40 μg/kg GRAN = 0.15 mg/kg x 3 OND	
328	≥70	GRAN 40 μg/kg iv	48		20
331		OND 0.15 mg/kg x 3 iv	51		
483	≥50	OND 8 mg iv + DEX 20 mg iv	79.3	OND + DEX = GRAN + DEX	21
483		GRAN 3 mg iv + DEX 20 mg iv	79.9		

C.P. = complete protection from vomiting; DOL = dolasetron; OND = ondansetron; GRAN = granisetron; DEX = dexamethasone

pimazine was shown to be significantly superior to ondansetron alone (complete protection from vomiting in 77.7% and 50% of patients, respectively) [23]. This study could suggest that the 5-HT_3 receptor complements (rather than replaces) the D_2 receptor.
The addition of metopimazine to the combination of ondansetron plus dexamethasone vs ondansetron plus dexamethasone needs to be evaluated in a very large patient population.

Are there new classes of antiemetics foreseen in the near future?

A new class of antiemetic agents could come from compounds acting at opiate receptors. In fact, in recent years there is growing evidence suggesting a role for opiate receptors (particularly μ receptors) in the emetic reflex arc. High densities of μ recognition sites were shown in the area postrema, nucleus tractus solitarius, dorsal motor nucleus of the vagus and reticular medulla in an autoradiographic study [24].
Morphine can influence emesis in a complex way, in particular, it can have both an emetic and an antiemetic effect. Either of these are antagonised by naloxone, indicating that both effects are mediated by opioid receptors. However, whereas the emesis is probably mediated by the area postrema, the antiemetic effects may occur in the "vomiting centre" [25]. Recently, naloxone has been shown to produce a dose-related increase in nausea and vomiting to cancer chemotherapy in paediatric patients, while the infusion of naloxone alone had no effect [26]. This observation suggests that a net inhibitory opiate effect, presumably acting at the level of the vomiting centre, is operative in the setting of cancer chemotherapy. Naloxone blocks this inhibitory effect and thereby increases nausea and vomiting in a dose-related fashion. It follows that exogenous opiates might increase the net inhibitory effect of endogenous opiates acting on the vomiting centre and therefore decrease chemotherapy-induced vomiting.
In another study, fentanyl, a highly potent μ receptor agonist, prevented the emesis induced by morphine, apomorphine, copper sulphate and cisplatin in the ferret. This antagonistic activity was inhibited by naloxone [25].
It is likely that in the near future effective antiemetic drugs can be developed which act at the μ receptor and can be devoid of the μ agonist-related activity on respiratory, cardiovascular and behavioural systems characteristic of morphine and fentanyl.
Other interesting receptors probably involved in the emesis induced by cancer chemotherapy are the 5-HT_{1A} receptors. The use of bus-

pirone (a partial agonist at $5HT_{1A}$ receptors with weak dopamine antagonist activity when used at higher doses) or 8-OH-DPAT (a selective agonist at $5\text{-}HT_{1A}$ receptors) suppressed vomiting induced by cisplatin, motion, and xylazine (which elicits vomiting by stimulating α-2-noradrenergic receptors) in the cat [27-28]. Their antiemetic effect is likely to be due to an action at a convergent structure, presumably at or near the vomiting centre. At present, no clinical data are available on the antiemetic activity of the agonists of $5\text{-}HT_{1A}$ receptors.

Other new classes of antiemetic drugs that seem foreseeable in the near future are the use as an antiemetic of an old anaesthetic drug, propofol, and the NK_1 receptor antagonists. In fact, sub-hypnotic doses of propofol possess direct antiemetic properties in postoperative nausea and vomiting [29]. In a recent small pilot study in cisplatin recipients who failed antiemetic treatment with $5\text{-}HT_3$ antagonists plus dexamethasone, the addition of propofol increased the number of patients free from vomiting in the first 24 hours after chemotherapy [30]. Further controlled studies are needed to confirm these preliminary results.

Recently, basic research has introduced the possibility that Substance P may be responsible for emesis induced by chemotherapy. In fact, the nucleus tractus solitarius has been shown to contain vagal afferent fibres that are innovated by Substance P and a Substance P receptor antagonist selective for human type NK_1 receptors (CP-99,994) has been shown to attenuate retching and vomiting induced by cisplatin in the ferret [31-32].

Phase I-II studies in humans are awaited with interest.

The Unsatisfactory Control of Delayed Emesis

Despite the great achievements in the control of acute emesis obtained in recent years, one is more and more aware of the shortcomings in the prevention of delayed emesis.

A recent study showed that despite the application of the combination of metoclopramide plus dexamethasone (the "standard" treatment) [33-34] about 50% of patients still suffer from delayed vomiting and/or nausea during days 2 to 4 after cisplatin chemotherapy [35]. Furthermore, this study demonstrated that: 1) the incidence and the intensity of delayed emesis remained similar during 3 consecutive cycles of cisplatin chemotherapy; 2) the presence of delayed emesis in the prior cycle of chemotherapy influenced the acute and delayed emesis of the subsequent cycle; 3) high doses of cisplatin and poor control of acute emesis are the most important prognostic factors in causing delayed emesis. Unfortunately, the efficacy of $5\text{-}HT_3$ antagonists has not been clearly demonstrated for this indication.

Recently, the results of a double-blind study involving 767 patients in which ondansetron 8 mg bid for days 2 to 6 or for days 2 and 3 only was compared to placebo have been published in abstract form [36]. All patients received ondansetron 0.15 mg/kg every 4 hours for 3 doses for the control of acute emesis. In this study the patients receiving ondansetron (both on days 2 and 3 and on days 2 to 6) presented significantly fewer emetic episodes than those receiving the placebo, but the number of patients achieving complete protection from delayed emesis was not significantly different between active treatment and placebo (35% vs 25%).

Therefore, it seems that ondansetron has some efficacy with respect to placebo but the clinical relevance of this activity is, at best, moderate. The combination of corticosteroids with a $5\text{-}HT_3$ antagonist vs the standard metoclopramide plus corticosteroids is probably worthy of more accurate evaluation in the prevention of delayed emesis. However, in planning such studies one has to be aware that a revised definition of delayed emesis induced by cisplatin has recently been suggested [37].

In fact, in patients receiving for acute emesis placebo or metoclopramide or ondansetron, the course of emesis over the 24 hours following cisplatin administration seems characterised by two vomiting peaks: one at approximately 4 hours and one at 18 hours, with a period of virtually "no vomiting" between them even in patients receiving placebo. While both metoclopramide and ondansetron attenuate the first peak significantly, neither eliminates or attenuates the second peak at 18 hours.

These observations, which need confirmation in a large population, would suggest that the phenomenon of delayed emesis may begin at 16 hours rather than 24 hours.

A pilot study in 91 patients in which antiemetic prophylaxis for delayed emesis with ondansetron (8 mg every 8 h for 2 days) combined with dexamethasone (8 mg every 12 h for 2 days then 4 mg every 12 h for 2 further days) was started at 16 hours after cisplatin chemotherapy, achieved 67% complete protection [38].

The Identification of the Best Rescue Treatment

Despite the new achievements, approximately 5-10% of patients still suffer from acute severe nausea and/or vomiting and need rescue treatment [39]. Unfortunately, no data from controlled studies are available to suggest the most appropriate antiemetic regimen, although both 5-HT_3 antagonists and high-dose metoclopramide, often in combination with steroids, are being currently employed. The most serious obstacle in carrying out a study on this topic is the huge number of patients that would have to be monitored to assure the inclusion of a sufficient number of "treatment failures" in a randomised controlled trial.

Inadequate Antiemetic Efficacy During Subsequent Cycles of Chemotherapy

In almost all antiemetic studies the efficacy and tolerability of antiemetic drugs have been evaluated during only one cycle of chemotherapy. However, the few methodologically correct studies which evaluated the persistence of antiemetic efficacy during multiple cycles of chemotherapy showed a significant decrease in complete protection from acute vomiting, nausea and both nausea and vomiting with high-dose metoclopramide combinations [40]. With ondansetron plus dexamethasone there was a persistence of complete protection from vomiting during subsequent cycles, but the complete protection from nausea and both nausea and vomiting decreased, albeit at a lower degree than with metoclopramide combinations [41]. The causes of this phenomenon are unknown. Some evidence exists that documents a possible role of delayed emesis in this phenomenon. In fact, the presence of delayed emesis in the previous cycle may increase the probability of suffering from acute emesis in the subsequent cycles [35]. So far no particular strategies have been tested to reduce the incidence of this phenomenon.

The Identification of Optimal Dose/ Schedule of Available Compounds

Data available to date for most compounds are insufficient to identify the most efficacious, suitable, well-tolerated and cost-effective regimen for cisplatin-treated patients and even more for patients submitted to "high-dose chemotherapy" regimens. The problem has clinical and economic implications, but the published data are at best scanty and sometimes contradictory.

Recently, 4 large studies have re-evaluated the problem of the optimal dose and schedule of ondansetron [5-8]. In 2 double-blind studies [5,6] a single 32 mg intravenous dose of ondansetron administered before cisplatin showed similar efficacy and toxicity compared with an 8 mg loading dose followed by a 24-hour infusion of 1 mg/h.

One of these studies [6] involving 535 patients included a third treatment arm in which patients received only a single 8 mg intravenous dose before cisplatin chemotherapy. Control of emesis was similar in all 3 groups, with complete protection from vomiting in about 55% of patients. More recently, 8 mg i.v. and 32 mg i.v. single dose of ondansetron obtained similar results in another double-blind trial [8].

However, these results were not confirmed in a double-blind study evaluating 699 patients [7]. In fact, the efficacy of an 8 mg intravenous single dose of ondansetron or of 0.15 mg/kg every 4 hours x 3 intravenous doses was shown to be inferior to a 32 mg intravenous single dose.

Recently, the optimal dose of granisetron has been more precisely identified. Initial studies indicated 3 mg single dose i.v. of granisetron as the optimal dose, but two dose ranging studies did not show any statistically significant difference in efficacy between 10 µg/kg (1 mg) and 40 µg/kg (3 mg) [42-43]. However, they were small studies, and therefore able to demonstrate only very large differences between dosages. Moreover, in one of these studies 40 µg/kg gave numerically superior results to 10 µg/kg for complete protection from emesis, no more than 1 vomiting episode and the clinician's global assessment of efficacy [42].

A large trial presented at the 1995 American Society of Clinical Oncology meeting showed that 1 mg single dose i.v. is equivalent to 3 mg

single dose i.v. and should be considered the optimal dose of granisetron [20].
More studies are needed to clarify the optimal dose and schedule of ondansetron as well as the other 5-HT_3 compounds.

The Cost-Efficacy Analyses

The 5-HT_3 antagonists are expensive drugs with respect to the costs of high-dose metoclopramide regimens. At present, only a limited number of pharmacoeconomic analyses have been performed on 5-HT_3 antagonists (in particular ondansetron) in the prevention of cisplatin-induced emesis and many of these are available only in abstract form [44]. These studies were based on a limited number of patients and pharmacoeconomic analysis was based mostly on estimates.
Recently, a retrospective pharmacoeconomic analysis referring to a clinical trial enrolling a large population of patients submitted to ondansetron plus dexamethasone or metoclopramide plus dexamethasone plus diphenhydramine for 3 consecutive cycles of cisplatin chemotherapy has been published [45]. Calculated costs, although retrospectively estimated, were produced on the basis of a time and motion study to reduce the uncertainty of estimates as much as possible. This study demonstrated that despite the higher acquisition cost for ondansetron vs metoclopramide, the ondansetron regimen costs per patient decreased substantially when all direct hospital costs were taken into account (from 5.23-fold higher to 2.43, 2.23 and 1.82-fold higher at first, second and third cycle of chemotherapy, respectively). More problematic is the evaluation of comparative cost/efficacy ratio among the 5-HT_3 antagonists. In fact, major differences exist in their acquisition cost but the evaluation of cost of therapy with each compound is complicated by the variability in dosage and schedules employed.

Moderately Emetogenic Chemotherapy

The problems still needing a more satisfactory solution are similar to those encountered with highly emetogenic chemotherapy. We will focus our attention on the areas where there is a greater need for improvement. These are: 1) the control of acute emesis for chemotherapy regimens including cyclophosphamide, anthracyclines and carboplatin; 2) the control of delayed emesis; 3) the persistence of antiemetic activity in subsequent cycles of chemotherapy; 4) the control of emesis due to some form of chemotherapy.

Improve the Control of Acute Emesis

The main problem here is the finding that the relative efficacy of different antiemetic drugs (5-HT_3 receptor antagonists, steroids, metoclopramide) varies according to the type of chemotherapy given.
The acute emesis following cyclophosphamide (≥600 mg/m^2), doxorubicin (≥50 mg), carboplatin (≥300 mg/m^2) and epi-doxorubicin (≥75 mg/m^2) when used alone or in combination is generally prevented in 60%-80% of patients using steroids or a 5-HT_3 antagonist. To date, only two comparative double-blind trials have been published comparing a 5-HT_3 antagonist with dexamethasone [18,46]. In the first study [46] on 112 patients receiving intravenous anthracycline and/or cyclophosphamide and/or etoposide, dexamethasone was shown to have similar efficacy to ondansetron in the prevention of acute emesis but was superior in the control of delayed nausea. Both antiemetic regimens were well tolerated. On this basis, many authors suggested that in the prevention of acute emesis induced by moderately emetogenic drugs, the 5-HT_3 antagonists, although as efficacious as dexamethasone, are indicated only in those patients refractory to corticosteroids or in those who cannot use them. The second study [18], a double-blind study including 408 patients submitted to moderately emetogenic chemotherapy (cyclophosphamide 600-1000 mg/m^2, doxorubicin ≥50 mg/m^2, epirubicin ≥75 mg/m^2 or carboplatin ≥300 mg/m^2, used alone or in some combination), a combination of granisetron and dexamethasone has been compared with granisetron alone and dexamethasone alone. This study confirms that granisetron and dexamethasone have similar efficacy in the prevention of acute emesis and that patients who received granisetron had less protection from delayed vomiting and nausea than those who received dexamethasone alone. Furthermore, their combination was

shown to be superior to the two drugs used alone, achieving 92.6% and 71.9% complete protection from vomiting and nausea, respectively. Whether similar results could be obtained with other 5-HT_3 compounds or with a different dose and/or schedule remains to be seen.

For acute emesis induced by moderately emetogenic drugs the combination of 5-HT_3 antagonists with drugs other than corticosteroids also seems worthy of further study. In fact, in a small double-blind crossover study in patients receiving non-cisplatin chemotherapy who had vomited during previous cycles of chemotherapy, ondansetron plus metopimazine was shown to be more efficacious than ondansetron alone [47]. These results necessitated validation in larger controlled studies.

Control of Delayed Emesis

No specific antiemetic trials have been performed on the prevention of delayed emesis in this group of patients and therefore, although the incidence of this phenomenon is clearly documented with some antineoplastic agents (i.e., carboplatin, cyclophosphamide) no clear recommendation can be given about treatment. Furthermore, in many oncological centres antiemetic drugs are used as prophylactic agents on the day of chemotherapy administration only and during the following days as rescue treatment in patients who presented emesis.

Inadequate Antiemetic Efficacy During Subsequent Cycles of Chemotherapy

Very limited data are available on the persistence of the antiemetic activity during subsequent cycles of chemotherapy in patients submitted to moderately emetogenic drugs. In 107 breast cancer patients receiving 6 courses of adjuvant FAC chemotherapy and submitted to methylprednisolone plus thyethylperazine a continuous decrease in complete protection from vomiting from the first to the sixth cycle of chemotherapy was shown [48]. No data from well-conducted studies are at present available for steroids, 5-HT_3 antagonists or their combination.

Problems Related to Low Repeated Doses of Cisplatin

In patients receiving cisplatin at low, repeated doses (20-40 mg/m^2 x 4-5 day), two studies showed that the addition of steroids to ondansetron increased the antiemetic activity [49,50]. Overall, about 50%-60% of patients obtained complete protection from vomiting during days 1-5. Antiemetic efficacy in both studies was more evident in the first 2-3 days, with a decrease in efficacy occurring on the fourth and fifth days of chemotherapy. This is in direct opposition to the pre-ondansetron period, when the most severe nausea and vomiting occurred during the first days of chemotherapy (tolerance effect).

Therefore, some problems are still unsolved: 1) to increase the complete protection during the overall 5 days of chemotherapy; 2) to optimise dose and duration of corticosteroids (only the first 2 days or for the whole duration of chemotherapy?); 3) to evaluate the rate of nausea and vomiting on the days after chemotherapy interruption.

Conclusion

Despite the great improvement in the control of chemotherapy-induced emesis in cancer patients documented in many clinical trials, it is clear that such amelioration has not affected all patients and has not been found for all chemotherapy regimens. Furthermore, it is unknown if the results obtained in clinical trials are transferable to daily practice.

The effectiveness of the new antiemetic strategies needs more careful evaluation, and only when such data will be available will it be possible to identify more precisely the unmet needs of patients submitted to emetogenic chemotherapy. In the meantime, hopefully, research will provide new drugs and a better knowledge of the old ones to provide more effective answers to the problems brought to our attention.

REFERENCES

1 Del Favero A, Roila F, Tonato M: Reducing chemotherapy-induced nausea and vomiting. Current perspectives and future possibilites. Drug Safety 1993 (9):410-428

2 Andrews PL, Bhandari P, Davey PT, Bingham S, Marr HE, Blower PR: Are all 5-HT3 receptor antagonists the same? Eur J Cancer 1992 (28A Suppl1):2-6

3 Freeman AJ, Cunningham KT, Tyers MB. Selectivity of 5-HT3 receptor antagonists and anti-emetic mechanisms of action. Anti-Cancer Drugs 1992 (3): 79-85

4 Marr HE, Davey PT, Bartlett AJ: Emerging differences between 5-HT3 receptor antagonists. Anti-Cancer Drugs 1991 (2):513-518

5 Marty M, d'Allens H, et le Groupe Multicentrique Francais: Etude randomisée en double-insu comparant l'efficacité de l'ondansetron selon deux modes d'administration: injection unique et perfusion continue. Cahiers Cancer 1990 (2):541-546

6 Seynaeve C, Schuller J, Buser K, Porteder H, Van Belles, Sevelda P, Christmann D, Schmidt M, Kitchener H, Paes D, De Mulder PHM on behalf of the Ondansetron Study Group: Comparison of the anti-emetic efficacy of different doses of ondansetron, given as either a continuous infusion or a single intravenous dose, in acute cisplatin-induced emesis. A multicentre, double-blind, randomised, parallel group study. Br J Cancer 1992 (66):192-197

7 Beck TM, Hesketh PJ, Madajewicz S, Navari RM, Pendergrass K, Lester EP, Kish JA, Murphy WK, Hainsworth JD, Gandara DR, Bricker LJ, Keller AM, Mortimer J, Galvin DV, House KW, Bryson JC: Stratified, randomized, double-blind comparison of intravenous ondansetron administered as a multiple-dose regimen versus two single-dose regimens in the prevention of cisplatin-induced nausea and vomiting. J Clin Oncol 1992 (10):1969-1975

8 Ruff P, Paska W, Goedhals L, Pouillart P, Rivière A, Vorobiof D, Bloch B, Jones A, Martin C, Brunet R, Butcher M, Forster J, McQuade B, on behalf of the Ondansetron and Granisetron Emesis Study Group: Ondansetron compared with granisetron in the prophylaxis of cisplatin-induced acute emesis: a multicentre double-blind, randomised, parallel-group study. Oncology 1994 (51):113-118

9 Noble A, Bremer K, Goedhals L, Cupissol D, Dilly SG: A double-blind, randomised, crossover comparison of granisetron and ondansetron in 5-day fractionated chemotherapy: assessment of efficacy, safety and patient preference. Eur J Cancer 1994 (30A):1083-1088

10 Mantovani G, Macciò A, Curreli L, Bianchi A, Gebbia V, Testa A: Comparison of the effectiveness of three 5-HT3 receptor antagonists in the prophylaxis of acute vomiting induced by highly emetogenic chemotherapy (high-dose cisplatin) for treatment of primary head and neck cancer. Proc Am Soc Clin Oncol 1994 (13):428

11 Martoni A, Angelelli B, Guaraldi E, Strocchi E, Pannuti F: Granisetron vs ondansetron in the prevention of cisplatin-induced emesis. An open randomised cross-over study. Proc Am Soc Clin Oncol 1994 (13):431

12 Jantunen IT, Kataja VV, Johansson RT: Ondansetron and tropisetron with dexamethasone in the prophylaxis of acute vomiting induced by non-cisplatin-containing chemotherapy. Acta Oncologica 1992 (31):573-575

13 Bonneterre J, Hecquet B, on behalf of the French Northern Oncology Group: Granisetron iv compared with ondansetron iv plus tablets in the prevention of nausea and vomiting induced by a moderately emetogenic chemotherapy regimen: a randomized cross-over study. Presented at a Satellite to the 7th European Conference of Clinical Oncology and Cancer Nursing, Jerusalem, Israel (abstract book). Adelphi Communication, Macclesfield, UK 1993 pp 22-24

14 Jantunen IT, Muhonen TT, Kataja VV, flander MK, Teerenhovi L: 5-HT3 receptor antagonists in the prophylaxis of acute vomiting induced by moderately emetogenic che motherapy - a randomised study. Eur J Cancer 1993 (29A):1669-1672

15 Campora E, Simoni C, Rosso R: Tropisetron versus ondansetron nella prevenzione e controllo dell'emesi in pazienti sottoposte a chemioterapia con FAC/FEC per carcinoma mammario metastatico o operato. Minerva Medica 1994 (85):25-31

16 Massidda B, Laconi S, Foddi MR, Salamah K, Ionta MT: Prevention of non-cisplatin induced emesis: role of the antagonists of 5-HT3 receptors. Ann Oncol 1994 (5) Suppl.8:204

17 Gebbia V, Cannata G, Testa A, Curto G, Valenza R, Cipolla C, Latteri MA, Gebbia N: Ondansetron versus granisetron in the prevention of chemotherapy-induced nausea and vomiting. Cancer 1994 (74): 1945-1952

18 The Italian Group for Antiemetic Research: Dexamethasone, granisetron, or both for the prevention of nausea and vomiting during chemotherapy for cancer. New Engl J Med 1995 (332):1-5

19 Navari R, Hesketh T, Grote M, Cramer M, Law R, Whitmore J, Hahne W: A double-blind randomized, comparative iv study of single dose dolasetron vs ondansetron in preventing cisplatin-related emesis. Proc ASCO 1995 (14):522

20 Ritter H, Hall J, Mailliard J, Navari R, Friedman C, on behalf of the Granisetron Study Group: A comparative clinical trial of granisetron and ondansetron in the prophylaxis of cisplatin-induced emesis. Proc ASCO 1995 (14):528

21 Roila F, De Angelis V, Cognetti F, Ricci S, Contu A, Nuzzo A, Picece V, Buzzi F, Clerico M, Tonato M: Ondansetron vs granisetron, both combined with dexamethasone in the prevention of cisplatin-induced emesis. Proc ASCO 1995 (14):523

22 Baltzer L, Kris MG, Tyson LB, Rigas JR, Pisters KMW: The addition of ondansetron to the combination of metoclopramide, dexamethasone, and lorazepam did not improve vomiting prevention in patients receiving high-dose cisplatin. Cancer 1994 (73):720-723

23 Herrstedt J, Handberg J, Sigsgaard T, Hansen M, Dombernowsky P: Randomized, double-blind cross-over trial of the antiemetic effect and tolerability of ondansetron (OND) vs OND plus the dopamine D2

antagonist metopimazine in patients receiving platinum-based chemotherapy. 6th International Symposium on Supportive Care in Cancer, March 2-5, New Orleans, 1994 P-63*

24 Barnes NM, Bunce KT, Naylor RJ, Rudd JA: The actions of fentanyl to inhibit drug-induced emesis. Neuropharmacology 1991 (30):1073-1083

25 Costello DJ and Borison HL: Naloxone antagonizes narcotic self-blockade of emesis in the cat. J Pharmacol Exp Ther 1977 (203):222-230

26 Kobrinsky NL, Pruden PB, Cheang MS, Levitt M, Bishop AJ, Tenenbein M: Increased nausea and vomiting induced by naloxone in patients receiving cancer chemotherapy. Am J Ped Hem/Onc 1988 (10):206-208

27 Lucot JB and Crampton GH: 8-OH-DPAT suppresses vomiting in the cat elicited by motion, cisplatin or xylazine. Pharmacology Biochemistry & Behavior 1989 (33):627-631

28 Lucot JB and Crampton GH: Buspirone blocks cisplatin-induced emesis in cats. J Clin Pharmacol 1987 (27):817-818

29 Borgeat A, Wilder-Smith OHG, Saiah M, Rifat K: Subhypnotic doses of propofol possess direct antiemetic properties. Anesth Analg 1992 (74):539-541

30 Borgeat A, Wilder-Smith OHG, Wilder-Smith CH, Forni M, Suter PM: Adjuvant propofol for refractory cisplatin-associated nausea and vomiting. Lancet 1992 (340):679-680

31 Tattersall FD, Rycroft W, Hargreaves RJ: The tachykinin NK1 receptor antagonist CP-99,994 attenuates cisplatin induced emesis in the ferret. Eur J Pharmacol 1993 (259): r5-6

32 Tattersall FD, Rycroft W, Hill RG: Enantioselective inhibition of apomorphine-induced emesis in the ferret by the neurokinin, receptor antagonist CP-99,994. Neuropharmacology 1994 (33):259-260

33 Kris MG, Gralla RJ, Tyson LB, Clark RA, Cirrincione C, Groshen S: Controlling delayed vomiting: double-blind, randomized trial comparing placebo, dexamethasone alone, and metoclopramide plus dexamethasone in patients receiving cisplatin. J Clin Oncol 1989 (7):108-114

34 Moreno I, Rosell R, Abad A, Barnadas A, Carles J, Ribelles N, Solano V, Font A: Comparison of three protracted antiemetic regimens for the control of delayed emesis in cisplatin-treated patients. Eur J Cancer 1992 (28A):1344-1347

35 Italian Group for Antiemetic Research: Cisplatin-induced delayed emesis: Pattern and prognostic factors during three subsequent cycles. Ann Oncology 1994 (5):585-589

36 Navari R, Madajewicz S, Anderson N, Tchekmedyian N, Whaley W, Garewal H, Beck T, Anderson E, Liddle R, Ossi M: Oral ondansetron effectively controls cisplatin-induced delayed emesis. Proc ASCO 1995 (14):523

37 Kris MG, Pisters KMW, Hinkley L: Delayed emesis following anticancer chemotherapy. Support Care Cancer 1994 (2):297-300

38 Rittenberg CN, Gralla RJ, Lettow LA, Cronin MD, Kardinal CG: New approaches in preventing delayed emesis: altering the time of regimen initiation and use of combination therapy in a 109 patient trial. Proc ASCO 1995 (14):526

39 Roila F, Tonato M, Ballatori E, Del Favero A: Prevention of cisplatin-induced emesis. Lancet 1992 (340):972

40 Roila F, Tonato M, Basurto C, Picciafuoco M, Bracarda S, Donati D, Malacarne P, Monici L, Di Costanzo F, Patoia L, Ballatori E, Tognoni G, Del Favero A: Protection from nausea and vomiting in cisplatin-treated patients: high-dose metoclopramide combined with methylprednisolone versus metoclopramide combined with dexamethasone and diphenhydramine: a study of the Italian Oncology Group for Clinical Research. J Clin Oncol 1989 (7): 1693-1700

41 Italian Group for Antiemetic Research: Difference in persistence of efficacy of two antiemetic regimens on acute emesis during cisplatin chemotherapy. J Clin Oncol 1993 (11):2396-2404

42 Riviere A, on behalf of the Granisetron Study Group: Dose finding study of granisetron in patients receiving high-dose cisplatin chemotherapy. Br J Cancer 1994 (69):967-971

43 Navari RM, Kaplan HG, Gralla RJ, Grunberg SM, Palmer R, Fitts D: Efficacy and safety of granisetron, a selective 5-hydroxytryptamine-3 receptor antagonist, in the prevention of nausea and vomiting induced by high-dose cisplatin. J Clin Oncol 1994 (12):2204-2210

44 Plosker GL and Milne RJ: Ondansetron: a pharmacoeconomic and quality of life evaluation of its antiemetic activity in patients receiving cancer chemotherapy. PharmacoEconomics1992 (2):285-301

45 Ballatori E, Roila F, Berto P, De Angelis V, Neri C,Olivieri A, Tonato M, Del Favero A: Cost and cost-effectiveness analysis of ondansetron versus metoclopramide regimens. A hospital perspective from Italy. PharmacoEconomics1994 (5):227-237

46 Jones AL, Hill AS, Soukop M, Hutcheon AW, Cassidy J, Kaye SB, Sikora K, Carney DN, Cunningham D: Comparison of dexamethasone and ondansetron in the prophylaxis of emesis induced by moderately emetogenic chemotherapy. Lancet 1991(338):483-487

47 Herrstedt J, Sigsgaard T, Boesgaard M, Jensen TP, Dombernowsky P: Ondansetron plus metopimazine compared with ondansetron alone in patients receiving moderately emetogenic chemotherapy. N Engl J Med 1993 (328):1076-1080

48 Martin M, Diaz-Rubio E, Casado A, Dominguez S, Sastre J: Progressive loss of antiemetic efficacy during subsequent courses of chemotherapy. Eur J Cancer 1992 (28):430-432

49 Weissbach L, Multi-day Cisplatin Emesis Study Group: Ondansetron. Lancet 1991 (338):753

50 Fox SM, Einhorn LH, Cox E, Powell N, Abdy A: Ondansetron versus ondansetron, dexamethasone and chlorpromazine in the prevention of nausea and vomiting associated with multiple-day cisplatin chemotherapy. J Clin Oncol 1993 (11):2391- 2395

www.ingramcontent.com/pod-product-compliance
Lightning Source LLC
Chambersburg PA
CBHW061216240926
51846CB00006B/1245
9783642802423